Understanding Weight Control

Understanding Weight Control

Mind and Body Strategies for Lifelong Success

Deborah C. Saltman, MD, PhD

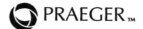 PRAEGER™

An Imprint of ABC-CLIO, LLC
Santa Barbara, California • Denver, Colorado

Library of Congress Cataloging-in-Publication Data

Names: Saltman, Deborah C., author.
Title: Understanding weight control : mind and body strategies for lifelong success / Deborah C. Saltman, MD.
Description: Santa Barbara, California : Praeger, an imprint of ABC-CLIO, LLC, [2018] | Includes bibliographical references and index.
Identifiers: LCCN 2017044438 (print) | LCCN 2017047066 (ebook) | ISBN 9781440857218 (ebook) | ISBN 9781440857201 (print : alk. paper)
Subjects: LCSH: Weight loss—Physiological aspects—Popular works. | Weight loss—Psychological aspects—Popular works.
Classification: LCC RM222.2 (ebook) | LCC RM222.2 .S2365 2018 (print) | DDC 613.2/5—dc23
LC record available at https://lccn.loc.gov/2017044438

ISBN: 978-1-4408-5720-1 (print)
     978-1-4408-5721-8 (ebook)

22 21 20 19 18   1 2 3 4 5

This book is also available as an eBook.

Praeger
An Imprint of ABC-CLIO, LLC

ABC-CLIO, LLC
130 Cremona Drive, P.O. Box 1911
Santa Barbara, California 93116-1911
www.abc-clio.com

This book is printed on acid-free paper ∞
Manufactured in the United States of America

This book discusses treatments (including types of medication and mental health therapies), diagnostic tests for various symptoms and mental health disorders, and organizations. The authors have made every effort to present accurate and up-to-date information. However, the information in this book is not intended to recommend or endorse particular treatments or organizations, or substitute for the care or medical advice of a qualified health professional, or used to alter any medical therapy without a medical doctor's advice. Specific situations may require specific therapeutic approaches not included in this book. For those reasons, we recommend that readers follow the advice of qualified health care professionals directly involved in their care. Readers who suspect they may have specific medical problems should consult a physician about any suggestions made in this book.

Contents

Preface

"Who are you writing this book for?" asked my best friend, who is also named Debra and who was the inspiration for this book. Debra had lost a total of 60 lb over four years through a variety of disruptive measures and was still losing more weight.

On that day, she was amazed—and maybe amused—by what I had just done.

A clinical physician who's authored 10 books and has developed an expertise in weight management, I was, at the time of that conversation, a size 10 and had been for more than a decade. But I still felt like a size 18. We were on vacation, and I had just thrown out a perfectly good sweater because I thought the horizontal stripes on it made me look fat.

I actually said that out loud.

It wasn't looking in the mirror that was the angst-invoking challenge; it was the memory of me at size 18 wearing clothes with horizontal stripes.

But things have changed now, years later.

Memories of when I was a heavyweight only make me proud today of how much I have changed. It wasn't easy, and my weight management will certainly be a never ending, lifelong quest. But it's a worthwhile venture. I am happy.

So, for whom is this book written? For people like me, who despise what their scales say or said and who, whatever our weight, always tend to see ourselves as fat. I hope sharing my story and the stories of people I have assisted will provide an ongoing, always helpful resource for everyone who reads it, an inspiration for every overweight or obese person seeking a long-term approach to weight loss.

Hopefully, this will be the one book about overweight and obesity on your Kindle, iPad, or bookshelf that is a "keeper."

Acknowledgments

This book is dedicated to my family, in particular to my best friend, expert critic, and lovely sister Dr. Maureen Waine and to my wonderful brother-in-law Dr. Eric Waine. We have all struggled with weight together.

Many willing minds have helped me along the way—both expert patients and expert clinicians. Thank you all. Here are just a few whom I can name: Natalie O'Dea, who helped me find the first ingredients, and Samantha Joel, a talented chef who taught me to cook up any number of different weight-loss diets. Of course, there is always a support team—Professors Monika Thomas and Michael Kidd, Dr. Inge Okkes, Chris Moller, and Joan Fitzhenry—who never lost faith in my abilities.

Special thanks to Professor Julie Silver, who gave me the skills to write such a complex book, and to Debbie Carvalko, the most wonderful editor a writer could have, and to the production team: Bridget Austiguy-Preschel, Nitesh Sharma, and Fred Dahl.

Introduction

Obesity is not one disease but a number of interconnected diseases and problems that come about through the interaction between our genetic makeup and our environment. It runs in families. Between 25 and 40% of our weight is determined by our genes and what goes on in our cells. Genes influence not only the ways we take in nutrients and excrete them but also the way we store our fat. The rest of our predisposition to fat is dictated by environmental factors, such as our access to unhealthy food, the portion sizes we eat, and the ways we may use food as an emotional crutch.

"Obesity" and "overweight" are often used interchangeably because the same health risks are attached to both of them. I prefer to use the term "overweight," which gives us an understanding that our weight is modifiable and relegates "obesity" to the extreme end of too much weight, often where drastic surgical intervention is necessary to achieve real change.

The degree of risk is greater the more overweight or obese we are. Body mass index (BMI) is the current measurement used to determine whether we are overweight or obese. BMI is calculated by dividing our weight in kilograms (kg) divided by our height in meters squared (m^2). The normal range for BMI is 18.5–24.9; overweight is 25–29.9; obese is 30.0–39.9; and extreme obese is ≥ 40.

To calculate your own BMI, The Centers for Disease Control and Prevention has an easy-to-use BMI calculator (Adult BMI Calculator).[1]

Changing our weight involves a lot of measuring to see how we progress; for example, we measure our weight, the calories (energy content) of what we eat, how long we undertake physical activity, and so on. The units used for the measurements depend on which side of the Atlantic you live. In the United States, ounces, pounds, inches, feet, and calories are the common measurements. However, a lot of the research is conducted in kilograms, grams, centimeters, meters, joules. It may be confusing, especially when reading articles or checking food content, so I have tried to include both sets of measurements here, wherever possible.

Those reading this book have most likely lost weight at least once in their lives and have probably also bought several books and read hundreds of articles on weight loss, so they will be familiar with some of the terminology. We know that losing weight in the first place is not usually the main problem. No matter what we do, any proven weight-loss program will help us to lose at least 5–10% of our weight in the first six months. Up to 90% of us maintain that weight loss for between six and 12 months—but it doesn't last. That is why weight loss is big business—because so many of us need continual help to keep the weight off.

> *Up to 50% of dieters who reduce their weight to a healthy level put weight back on within five years, and the more we lose, the more likely most of us are to regain it.*

Everybody knows how to get weight off. That doesn't necessarily mean eating less. What it means is eating a balanced diet of nutritional foods and burning up more calories than you take in. One step at a time, one day at a time. But the strategies we use to lose weight are usually not sustainable. Dieting gets boring, and so do the same exercises day after day, and we can pay only so much attention to them in our very busy days. Besides, we really do have bodies that are programmed to put on weight.

The problem with all weight-loss programs is that they are designed for the short term. None really deliver in the long term, that is, the term of our natural lives. That's because the constellation of complex problems that cause obesity have grown slowly in our minds as well as in our bodies, and they require a range of lifelong strategies to manage.

> *Obesity is not a disease that can be "cured." It is a lifelong challenge that requires a lot of disruption of our old ways in the beginning and a lifetime of managing change.*

For many of us, the lifetime plan seems like a daunting battle. Even just taking 30 to 60 minutes a day to do each of the dozen or so proven techniques like diet planning, exercise, and psychological commitment may seem as though it would leave little free time for thinking about anything else. But sustainable healthy weight requires attention to a range of activities, including diets, at different times. The idea that we can tackle everything all at once is not workable and is a flaw of current short- and medium-term thinking. Hence, weight loss demands time and attention, but it is time and attention well spent to better the rest of your life.

Certainly, we do have to establish healthy routines to lose weight. And once something becomes "routine," it is—or at least seems to be—less time-consuming. But just as our minds usually lose motivation after prolonged activity of many kinds, our bodies may refuse to lose weight if left too long on the same restrictive diet or exercise regimen. Sports enthusiasts of many types, including bodybuilders, call this kind of halt to the intended results even while continuing an eating and exercise routine "hitting a wall." The sought-after effect stops for no obvious reason.

Weight loss is a continuing challenge, for both our minds and our bodies. Reading about the latest fad doesn't help. A dizzying number of "tried-and-tested" remedies are on offer in the 200-plus research articles published on weight-related issues every day: drugs, physical activity, low-calorie/low-fat diet, regular breakfast, self-confidence, commitment to lifelong change, therapeutic alliances with clinicians, long-term self-help groups, face-to-face/Web-based interventions, and more. Some people just get desperate and try anything, and when nothing seems to work, they relapse into their old ways.

What we need to do is on the same plane as what those bodybuilders do to control their weight when they "hit the wall"—vary their diet and their exercise. It's a key to control, whether one is trying to gain or lose weight. There is no miracle solution to buy. The "magic" is in having the self-control to create excitement and variety, so that your mind doesn't get bored and your body won't acclimate.

Most of us want to believe there is some miracle cure that we can buy and that will end our suffering once and for all. There isn't one. Media attract our attention, especially on quiet news days, with terms like "breakthrough," "miracle," "cure," "revolutionary," and similar attention-getting words. Thirty-six new drugs associated with losing weight used these terms in press releases in one year. Half of them hadn't even been approved by the FDA, and five were "groundbreaking" only in mice or test tubes. When "promising" or "breakthrough" are added to a facts-only description of a drug, we are even more likely to believe it is going to be effective.[2] We need to challenge the obesity industry to come up with composite solutions that are sustainable. Right now all we have is a lot of short-term products with built-in obsolescence from an obese industry whose voracious goal is to feed a desperate market. The best we can do is to commit to change any strategy when it stops working for us and not see the change as a failure.

That is why I developed the weight disruption program.

Fortunately, it works. I am living proof, and so are my patients who are following my lead.

What Is Weight Disruption?

Most of the time, when we try to lose weight or maintain a healthy weight, our bodies (and minds) follow one of a series of set pathways to maintain our overweight state. Each of us has a weight range that is determined by our genes and that we are programmed to maintain. This natural weight range is called our "set-point." Our bodies' internal mechanisms keep our weight within this range. For example, our metabolism will work faster if we eat more than we need in order to maintain our set-point weight. Conversely, if we don't eat enough to maintain our weight, then our metabolism slows down and spares the available calories.[3] If we are predisposed to becoming overweight or obese, these mechanisms don't function properly.[4]

And our dysfunctional "fat" minds can contribute. We look in the mirror. We think we look fat, so we are ashamed. We get anxious. We get something to eat to make us feel better. Unfortunately, the destination of "feeling better" is not the last stop on this pathway. We travel on to feeling guilty that we ate, angry that we have "destroyed" all our previous good work, and too ashamed to talk with anyone about it. So we eat more.

Or a dysfunctional physical pathway may also switch on when we are trying lose weight, and we plateau, or hit the wall—usually at about three months. The hormones in our stomach start to work as if the diet is preventing us from getting enough calories to live. And the hormones work even harder to hang onto every calorie from food.

Disruptive weight management works to change these pathways—again and again, until they no longer are the pathways that our bodies and minds settle into. For me, disruptive weight management is a lifelong feel-good activity. I hope it becomes yours.

The process requires disrupting our bodies and minds from being comfortable with fat and in the long term rewires them. Designed for serious long-term losers, it is a technique that I have practiced and taught for over 20 years.

There are only four simple messages in weight disruption.

1. Disruption and rewiring are lifelong paths.

Rather than one particular strategy, disrupting our weight requires us to engage in a range of approaches and keep changing them until our minds and bodies no longer operate in comfortably fat mode. We need to upgrade frequently to reach and stay at our goals. For example, to start disruptive dieting, we need to accept that once the diet we have chosen isn't working anymore, we need to change it and use another strategy, not wait six months until we are blocked by a thick "wall of plateau," feel overwhelmed, lose ambition, have our next health crisis or panic, and fail at trying to prepare for an event where we want to look good.

2. As disrupters, we are unique and special.

Every weight management activity begins as a personal experiment and is a gift to ourselves. We are on our own adventure. We are our own specific researchers and advisors. Often, the approaches are quite different from general plans suggested by experts through years of interpreting and dispensing strategies that are not specific to us.

We are busy finding new strategies until both the shame and guilt about our weight no longer takes us down a destructive pathway of weight regain or inactivity. This may mean going against what we have been told. It may make it difficult for us to relate to those who want to help us but who are caught up in their conventional ways of thinking. For example, most experts will tell us that laxatives should not be used in a weight management program. That is not true. If you have a lapse and put on a few pounds, there is nothing wrong in using laxatives for a few days to get those few pounds off and get the lean engine running again.

3. Disruption takes time.

This process takes time because we want it to work lifelong. Usually, when we are ready for fat-disruptive techniques to begin, our bodies, minds, and support systems are strongly in defense of our fat mode. A complete change of fat mode to lean mode takes years. But just as we learned in primary school how to read and write and now we don't have to think about those tasks, weight disruption can become part of our lives. It has for me and for many of my patients.

4. Disruption must be accompanied by rewiring and new construction.

It is not enough to just disrupt our unhelpful thoughts and actions. We need to continually construct new ones and avoid reconstructing the old ones, such as the idea that we cannot tackle all that is needed at once for a prolonged period. We need to continually challenge our minds. Turning negative concepts into positive ones helps. "I've eaten a piece of cake. I've failed" can become "I've eaten a piece of cake. I must increase my physical activity today." At times, we will need the encouragement or help of others.

However, we must not get stuck on that need to have someone else telling us that change is okay. No one strategy works for a long time without some new constructing, with the most potentially intense being medical intervention or mental health therapy. Most of all, we need to tolerate our guilt, shame, and anxiety and diminish their power by embracing new ways of eating, being active, and thinking healthy.

Notes

1. https://www.cdc.gov/healthyweight/assessing/bmi/adult_bmi/english_bmi _calculator/bmi_calculator.html
2. https://thethinker.co/2015/11/11/transforming-crowdsourcing-into-thera peutic-advance
3. http://www.cci.health.wa.gov.au/docs/set%20point%20theory.pdf
4. http://mediendo.cn/uploadfiles/kejian/20140728/0728163529_1319.pdf# page=71

CHAPTER ONE

How and Why We Get Fat

We are learning more every day about how we get fat and how our bodies adapt, often poorly, to the fat that we gain. The reasons why we get fat are easily explained in simple language—our genes, our bodies, our environments—but the science behind those words is increasingly complex. Basically, we are what we got in our genes from both our mothers and fathers, what we absorbed in the way of nutrition and toxins in the womb, what we got rid of, and what we did as we grew up to indulge or moderate our bodies along the way.

This chapter goes into more depth about the science behind what we read in the newspapers and magazines about excessive weight and obesity. The main messages, however, are quite straightforward:

- There is a lot of hype about what "causes" us to become obese. Very little of what we read has good evidence—such as that watching television has been associated with obesity—and when it does, it is really only part of a much bigger, more complex picture. Television watching is not the problem; it is the eating and lack of physical activity that come with watching television that are problematic.

- It doesn't matter which method we use to measure how obese we are. They all work. Some are best for assessing what other health problems may accompany our obesity; for example, where the fat is situated on the body tells us a little about the risks to our heart. Then there are methods used by specialists to compare us with people in the general population and sometimes to determine what kind of treatments we can have. For instance, body mass index is used to decide whether we are suitable candidates for bariatric surgery. On a personal level, daily measurements such as weighing and clothes fit are useful as indicators of which direction we are heading—increasing, decreasing, or plateauing in weight.

- Obesity and overweight have complex beginnings, and their management involves a series of individualized and sequenced approaches. Treatments (or preventative efforts) need to be adapted and changed over time depending on how our disruption is going.[1] A cluster of strategies is often required for the cluster of problems.[2,3]

I was a fat kid. I was born "large" at 8 lb 6 oz. Well, that was large compared with my older sister who weighed just 6 lb at birth. I was part of the "lucky" generation—we had enough food, and we ate it. Sometimes my mother would say I was eating for the whole family to make up for how they starved as children. Until the age of 10, when my overweight grandmother had a stroke and couldn't cook anymore, I used to eat four meals a day plus snacks. At 8 a.m., mom would drop me off at school on her way to work, telling me I had to have a milk drink for my bones. Lunch was always healthy, but I usually traded it with my school friends for their little packets of sweets. I would go to my grandparents' house after school to wait for my parents to come from work. My grandmother always had a two-course meal prepared for me. In her strongly accented voice, I could hear how desperate she was to feed me. She had suffered through several wars and starved, and she didn't want that for her grandchildren. I felt guilty, so I ate everything on my plate, even if I felt full long before the plate was empty. Little did I know, my stomach and brain were then plotting a lifelong strategy to ensure I would never starve like my grandmother. And when my parents came home, my mother or father prepared another two-course meal.

I had a full package of causes to get fat—among them, survival genes, antistarvation signals in my mother's womb, and bad behavioral patterns of eating set up when I was young. A lifetime of energy intake over energy expenditure—eating more calories than I burned up with activities all day—was part of my programming. Over time, weight gain and obesity settled in my body and stayed. Managing my weight became my lifelong challenge.

It took me a long time to realize that how I got fat was important when I lost my motivation; knowing that helped me understand that I was not "to blame" or "helpless." I couldn't change the fact that my body developed an enormous capacity to store energy for bad times.

That capacity is mainly stored in adipose tissue, which consists of fat cells, or adipocytes. These cells are not just storage depots for energy but active hormonal glands, secreting hormones that can regulate our appetite and our body metabolism. Fat cells do much more than just affect how we look. Have you ever noticed how obese and overweight people wear less clothing than slender people, yet they often sweat more easily? That's because fat cells also are responsible for transforming chemical energy into heat.

Recently, scientists have discovered that not all fat cells are the same. In fact, some fat—fat that is brown in color—is good fat because it burns up energy. White fat is the worst fat. Its main function is to store excess energy and not use it. White fat cells are the most common fat cells in the body and are where the toxic excess weight is stored. Once this toxic fat is stored, it is hard to remove. We have to work on keeping these white fat cells as empty as possible of toxic fat. They are very efficient and can convert the energy from one piece of chocolate into a weight gain of 100 times the weight of that chocolate.

Originally, it was thought that we had only white fat cells and that they were there for life accumulating toxic fat. Now we know that white fat cells are more than waste dumps; they are active glands with hormones that control our eating patterns. More on this later.

Fortunately, some white fat cells can also be turned into fat-dissolving cells called "brite" (brown in white) or beige fat cells. These beige cells are found in pockets of white cells and can increase energy expenditure and potentially protect us against obesity and diabetes. Women have more active brown/beige fat than men.[4] We don't yet know how white fat cells turn beige, but we do know that, under conditions of high feeding, they can turn white again.[5]

The good news is that the old beliefs about fat cells are being challenged. It was previously thought that the only way to deal with toxic white fat cells was to keep them empty or have them removed surgically. Now we know that they can be triggered to work differently. Many new therapies for obesity are working on ways to turn these white cells into beige ones. Some of these experimental drugs are discussed in Chapter 10.

The most energy-efficient fat cells are brown fat cells. Unfortunately, they are less common than white fat cells. Brown fat is usually found around muscles, especially in the neck, inner chest, kidney, and spinal regions. In newborn babies, brown fat is also found between the shoulder blades. Whereas white fat just stores energy, brown fat gets rid of it—usually by converting it into heat. Brown fat is like our internal fuel burner. Like central heating, brown fat gets more turned on in colder weather, especially in winter.[6] When fully activated, our body's brown fat cells can produce as much heat energy as 20 Olympic cyclists generate in cycling on the road. As little as 50 g (1.8 oz) of activated brown fat can increase our daily energy expenditure (calorie burn) by one-fifth and burn 4 kg (8.8 lb) of body fat per year.[7]

> *Our brown fat cells can pro-
> duce as much energy in a
> day as 20 Olympic triathletes
> burn in a minute.*[8]

So, although not all fat is unhealthy, many of us still confuse fat cells with how our body looks when gaining weight. Yet some fat is essential for my body to function; for example, cholesterol is the basis of our sex hormones. Fat above the minimal amount is referred to as "nonessential fat." The amount of nonessential fat varies between the sexes and with age. Women need 12%, and men need about 3% of their body weight in fat, but up to 20–32% of body weight for women and 10–22% for men is still compatible with health.[9] It is this nonessential fat that gives our bodies a healthy look—rounded and smooth skin. It also differentiates the male shape from the female shape.

When men put on nonessential fat, it generally accumulates around their middle—supposedly making them look like apples. With women, the fat is more likely to gather around the hips and thighs, supposedly making them look like pears. These kinds of distinctions aren't really helpful—nor are they always correct. Oprah and I have something in common, our fat was not in the traditional female places. My fat was up front, that is, in my breasts and abdomen—neither apple nor pear.

Body Shapes

The athletic, or mesomorphic, build is the most muscular shape. It is a shape that lots of us try very hard to achieve—especially men. Unfortunately, if you don't have that build from childhood, it is difficult to maintain it as an adult, and the muscle can be quickly replaced by fat. When you see elite athletes later in life, many of them have replaced their muscles with fat, Muhammad Ali, for example. When fat covers the whole body, and hides our muscles, it is called an endomorphic shape. Most people, like me, are a combination of these two body types. These combinations are more likely to be found in people with weight problems; for example, meso-morphic/endomorphic women like me are more likely to have more body weight and higher fat-to-muscle ratios with lower lean mass and water content than all other groups.

Sometimes we can mistake the appearance of a skinny body for having low muscle and low fat. This is not always the case. There is a type of body, the ectomorphic body, that has a slim build, with long limbs and narrow shoulders and hips. We have all seen these people and wondered how they keep the weight off. Though this shape appears lean, ectomorphs have both low body fat and low muscle mass and usually more fat than muscle, so they can be, relatively speaking, overweight.

Marcia

Marcia's parents did the best they could for her. The whole family was "big." They had no idea what weight Marcia should be and steadfastly believed that any "baby fat" would turn into "sexy curves" at puberty. They had no scales in the house. None of them could see beyond their bellies to read what they weighed, anyway.

What might have been helpful for Marcia is some way of assessing or measuring her weight to see when it was getting out of control. Most treatment programs for obesity use some kind of measurement to assess the risk of her continuing on an obesity-bound pathway and, if she chose to deal with it, measuring her progress.

There are many ways to measure whether we are overweight or obese. Most of the criteria are based on a series of normal weight ranges for men—measurements taken of returned servicemen after World War II. Reference measurements for women were added later—though I am not sure how they were generated. Servicemen were an easy population to identify and measure but they didn't really represent the general population and certainly not the U.S. population at the end of the twentieth century, who were much better fed and taller.

The taller we are, the more body volume we have to distribute our fat. That is why taller people can weigh more and be healthier than shorter people of the same weight. Height is an important factor in assessing whether we are overweight or obese. Body mass index (BMI) was developed as a way to ensure that our weight is appropriate for our height. It is now the accepted way of assessing whether we are in the right weight range for our height compared with others in our age range. BMI is calculated as a person's weight in kilograms (kg) divided by their height in meters squared (m^2).

For example, a 40-year-old woman who weighs 90 kg (198 lb) and is 1.60 m (5′3″) tall would have a BMI of 90 kg ÷ (1.60 m × 1.60 m) = 90 ÷ 2.56 = 35.

Unfortunately, there are several limitations to BMI as the best way to measure overweight or obesity. BMI cannot distinguish between fat and muscle, and muscle is much heavier than fat. So people with large, bulky muscles—bodybuilders, for example—may have BMIs that are incorrectly classified as obese or overweight. Similarly, children's height and weight and the rate at which they put on weight and store it can vary a lot as a result of normal growth and development. While there are normal ranges for BMI in children that vary with age and sex, the calculations for any one child can vary a lot over the years.[10]

Muscle weighs more than fat. So our weight may not change as we get fitter, even though there may be a great improvement in appearance.

The BMI of children is compared with other children in the same way as height is by ranges of percentage of children in the same group (called percentiles). To determine overweight or obesity, a child is compared with other children. Overweight children have a BMI between the 85th and the 95th percentiles of the normal range for their age and sex. Obese children have a BMI at or greater than 95th percentile for age and sex. Severe obesity in childhood is defined at a BMI at or greater than 120% of the 95th percentile.

Besides muscle-to-fat ratio, cultural differences, and childhood variations, there are other reasons that we can't yet explain to suspect that BMI might not tell the whole story. For example, some people have all the health problems associated with obesity—such as diabetes, high blood pressure, arthritis, and depression—but have normal weight. Conversely, there are obese individuals with no other health problems who have a BMI above 30 kg/m^2.[11]

These exceptions to the BMI ranges make it difficult to use BMI as an ongoing measurement of how we are going in our weight disruption journey, because our starting points are so variable but the ranges are very fixed; for example, we could start on the upper limit of overweight (29.9), lose 4.5 kg (10 lb), and still be in the overweight category for our height and age. So it is not surprising that ranges are interpreted differently by clinicians and the general public. Surveys suggest that 60% of men believe that a BMI greater than 28 is a sign of overweight. However, 30% of men with a BMI of 30–31 (i.e., the lower end of the obese range) consider their weight acceptable. Older women also think that a BMI of 30–31 is acceptable, whereas younger women view the upper part of the normal range of BMI as overweight.

Once we have established that we need to work on our weight, there are many other ways to assess ongoing changes in body weight and fat. Some methods are quite simple and have been around for a long time, such as scales. Other methods are quite new and technical such as bioelectrical impedance analysis. Like BMI, every method has its limitations and benefits.

Table 1.1 outlines some of the methods available and how useful I think they are for us to keep track of our weight disruption activities. Because abdominal fat is becoming more important as a predictor of health problems, I have added a column that identifies which techniques can assess fat in the dangerous abdominal region. (Fat around the abdomen usually means there is fat around our heart, which can cause serious problems such as heart attacks.)

An easy way of assessing change in weight is how our clothes fit us, that is, how loose or tight they are. Our first signs of weight loss may be an alteration in a belt notch or the looseness of how clothes fit at the waist. It is best measured using the same clothes or belts every time. If we increase our physical activity, clothes fit may be a better indication of "getting into shape" than simple weight or body mass index measures—especially as muscle weighs more than fat and our weight may not have changed but has been converted from unhealthy fat into healthy muscle.

Excess fat around the middle is recognized as signaling toxic fat depositing around our major organs such as the heart, liver, and pancreas. Increased waist circumference is associated with increased health risks in patients with BMIs over 25. The high-risk waist circumferences are greater than 102 cm (40 in.) for men and greater than 88 cm (35 in.) for women. The good news is that all weight-loss modalities are better at getting rid of this toxic fat than they are at getting rid of superficial fat.

Our weight fluctuates on a daily basis, and this shouldn't scare us. I measure my weight daily so I can stay calm about the fluctuations.

From birth until death, scales have traditionally been used to assess weight gain and loss. While it is easy to do, assessing weight using scales is okay as a rough measure of weight change. It doesn't give us an accurate measure of where the weight changes are occurring or whether we are losing fat or just water. Also, excess weight shown on the scale does not necessarily mean we have excess fat. For women, weight changes during the menstrual cycle can be quite large—up to a few pounds as more or less water is retained. There is also a lot of variability in using scales, so try to be as consistent as possible. Here are some tips:

*   Buy a reliable scale, large enough for you to read, and place it on a firm, even surface (e.g. tiles not carpet).

Table 1.1

Method	Cost	Ease and Access	Usefulness	Measures Abdominal Fat
Clothes fit	Low	Easy and always available	This is relatively easy measure if we use the same clothing every time we measure and the clothes don't change shape (e.g., shrink through washing).	Yes—but not very accurately—especially if you suffer from bloating
Scales	Low	Easy and cheap to purchase	Easy and as reliable as the model you buy, but they only measure weight and if you have a big protruding abdomen, you may not be able to get a set that you can read.	No
Height and weight—body mass index (BMI)	Low	Easy, using a number of apps or programs	It's the standard measure and good to mark your starting point, but it is not very useful along the path to weight disruption because the formula is complicated, and it takes a long time to register change.	No
Tape measure—circumferences	Low	Easy to use	Measurements need to be taken at exactly the same place every time and are useful only if we haven't any medical problems that cause our abdomens to expand, such as bloating.	Yes
Skin fold	Low	Usually done by clinicians or sports physiologists	Not very helpful in weight loss because the more accurate measurements are in locations with little fat (e.g., arms), and with major weight loss, it is difficult to distinguish between skin and fat. This type of measurement, often called "skinfold analysis," is mainly used by fitness professionals to estimate body fat for people who are fit and trying to increase their muscle bulk.[a]	Yes

Method	Level	Where	Description	During pregnancy
Bioelectrical impedance (BIA)	Moderate	Can be done by most scales these days	Not helpful for women who have a lot of female fat distribution (e.g. large breasts) or very obese people.	No
Ultrasound	Moderate	Usually done by clinicians	Not practical because it is available only in specialist clinics. Ultrasound is best for measuring small changes in the fat around our waists, in our abdomens, and around our organs. It is also used extensively in estimating the weight of fetuses. It can help to predict whether a baby will be born overweight. The period before birth is one of the key times for rapid weight gain.[b]	Yes
Density (through immersion in water)	Moderate	Usually done in research studies	Not practical because it is available only in specialist clinics.	No
Dual X-ray absorptiometry (DXA)	High	Usually done in research studies	Not practical because it is available only in specialist clinics.	No
Computed tomography (CT scan)/ magnetic resonance imaging (MRI)	High	Usually done in research studies	Not practical because it is available in only specialist clinics and means getting a dose of radiation that may be unnecessary.	No

a. https://www.ncsf.org/enew/articles/articles-skinfoldassessment.aspx

b. https://www.hindawi.com/journals/jobe/2013/280713

- Measure your weight at the same time of day every time (best in the morning as our intake of food and drink and excretion of urine and bowel movements can vary during the day).
- Wear the same clothing each time (preferably as little as possible). I always weigh myself after a shower or bath.
- Avoid weighing yourself the week around your period (for women) because water retention can change our weight by up to 10 pounds.
- Avoid weighing yourself for a few days after a long airplane flight. The lower pressurization in the cabin results in our retaining a lot of fluid that we lose over the next few days.

Bioelectrical impedance analysis (BIA), a very useful technique to measure how much of our body weight is fat, muscle, or water, is now available in combination with scales. I use a combined set of scales. The addition of a BIA reading helps me understand my progress day by day both in weight and in how much fat I am amassing. It is especially useful when I am increasing my physical activity because muscle weighs more than fat, and I need to make sure my weight gain is muscle. It is also useful to help me know when my weight changes due to water retention, such as around my periods or when I drink a lot of any type of fluid or eat salty foods that attract water and cause it to be retained longer than normal.

BIA measures fat by passing a very small current through our body. The current travels at different speeds through fat and muscle. Muscles contain large amounts of water and healthy salts, which conduct electric current well. Fat is very resistant to electric current. The larger the impedance (i.e., the measurement) is, the higher the fat content. Commercial and home measuring systems usually come in two forms: lying down or standing on bathroom-style scales, like the ones I have, with measuring electrodes built into the footplate. While it is more convenient to stand on scales to take a BIA measurement, the measurement is not as accurate as it mainly flows through the limbs and across the chest, so it does not take into account abdominal fat.[12]

Like all measures of obesity and overweight, BIA has several limitations. In addition to the reading changing according to the amount of fluid we drink or the phase of our menstrual cycle, BIA tends to underestimate fat in obese people and overestimate fat in women with large breasts. It is also not very useful in adolescents where the fat distribution can be variable.[13]

How Often Should We Measure Our Weight?

In our daily lives, we are always assessing our weight, whether it is through the clothes we wear or looking at our bodies during our daily routines. We measure our weight every day in one way or another—just not formally. We get used to assessing what we look like. The same is true for weight. The more familiar and comfortable we are at looking at measurements of our weight, the more control we can have over the changes. Our weight fluctuates on a daily basis, and this shouldn't scare us. Regular, frequent measuring should be used as a technique to disrupt our negative thinking about what we might find when we read the scales or BIA. After years of daily weighing, I am now comfortable reading the scales and dealing with what I see. Daily measurement also alerts us to—aside from water weight or menstrual cycle gains—adjustments we should consider before any gains get tougher to stop or to reverse.

Overall, any method we use to measure how obese we are is beneficial. They all work, just in different ways, and supply different information. Some are best for assessing what other health problems may accompany our obesity; for example, where the fat is situated tells us something about the risks to our heart. Others are used by specialists to compare us with people in the general population and to determine what kind of help we need or are entitled to; for instance, body mass index is used to decide whether we are candidates for surgery. On a daily basis, weighing and clothes fit are the most useful as indicators of which direction we are heading—increasing, decreasing, or plateauing in weight.

Bill and Toni

Bill (5'10" and 220 lb) is obese (BMI 31.6), and Toni (5'5" and 160 lb) is overweight (BMI 27.1). They like each other partly because they are large, and now, after a decade of disruptive weight loss, both are content to be at the lower end of overweight. In the beginning, they had a scale that talked to them because Bill couldn't see over his stomach to read his weight. Bill liked hearing the voice, but Toni found it a bit freaky. Now that Bill can see over his stomach, they have a scale that also measures bioelectrical impedance. Both of them measure their weight daily, so they can stay calm about fluctuations. Bill has found that if he measured his weight only once a week, and it happened that he measured it on a day when his weight was at a high point, he'd feel depressed. Daily weighing is good for him. If he finds that his weight has gone up a couple of pounds, he can immediately do something about it. He can disrupt quickly. Toni doesn't always look at her weight. Sometimes she looks at the percentage of fat in her body on that day. She finds that particularly useful at different times of the month because during her menstrual cycle, the amount of water she retains changes quite markedly.

Where Does Obesity Begin?

As we will be seeing throughout this book, the causes and remedies for obesity are complicated and subject to influences both inside the body and outside it. Obesity and overweight are not life sentences. They are not programmed into the body; even the factors that cause them can change. Lifelong studies suggest that genetic effects can be age specific. Different obesity-promoting genes may become active at different ages over the life span. So even if some of the discovered genes consistently promote obesity, other genetic influences may appear at different stages to counteract them.

Erica

Erica lived with her mother, father, and brother. Her body mass index (BMI) was at the 88th percentile based on age and gender norms, which placed her in the obese range. Most of her weight was around her lower abdomen and legs. Her mother was overweight, but her father and brother were not overweight. Erica had a few close friends whom she described as "skinny" but who were really in the overweight range. She was well accepted in the family, and her parents believed her weight problem came completely from the genes on her mother's side. She umpired on the softball team, but beyond that did not engage in regular physical activity. Erica weighed herself every other day, and if she hadn't lost any weight, she skipped breakfast that day. But when she was hungry, she did eat breakfast, and it usually consisted of high-calorie, low-nutrient foods. She said she couldn't help it. It was in her genes—all her mother's family members were fat.

Associating particular genes with obesity is commonplace today. Our genetic footprint can now tell a lot about the likelihood of any one of us acquiring a range of diseases, including cancer, heart disease, or diabetes. However, that is still only part of the picture; identifying genes is only one step. We have 3.0 billion pairs of molecules that make up our genes.

So far, 135 different genes have been linked with the likelihood of our becoming overweight or obese. Eighteen of them can be directly related to obesity, 43 to body weight, and 12 to the distribution of body fat. Given that height plays a key role in the calculation of BMI, it may be important to consider that more than 700 genes are involved in body height.[14] The influence of these genes on the actual development of obesity is quite variable. Twin studies give us the best evidence. Between 50 and 90% of the obesity seen in twins can be related to their genes. In families, the genetic influence ranges between 20 and 80%. Looking at the general population, the

100-plus genes most closely linked to obesity account for about 2% of the differences in weight.[15]

There are genes that affect the size of the meals we eat and how often we eat. The influence on portion size and meal frequency is about 50% greater for those of us possessing these genes. To a lesser extent, genes can influence our consumption of foods high in fat, sugar, and salt and even of healthy foods such as fruits and vegetables. These genes have twice the effect on men compared to women.

> *The causes and remedies for obesity are subject to influences both inside the body and outside it.*

Beyond Our Genetic Footprint for Obesity: Critical Growth Periods

There are *critical growth periods* in our lives when our potential to become fat can be accelerated: in the womb, before we start walking in early childhood, and adolescence. In each of these periods, different factors are at work, and many of these factors can be modified. For Erica, despite her genetic makeup, she still could work on these issues by disrupting what she was doing and developing a lifelong plan for healthy weight.

During pregnancy, our mothers adapt their metabolism to support our fetal growth and development. This happens in two phases. In the first two trimesters of pregnancy, our mothers are in more or less in a state of starvation because they are feeding two. Extra insulin in the body helps them store fat for later. In the third trimester, our mothers' bodies reject the insulin and the fat storage process, so that all the stored nutrients can be shunted to us as we get ready to be born.

It is paradoxical and strange to think that the weight gain that might be okay for our mother in the first two trimesters may be not okay in the third. It is the same whether our mothers are skinny, normal, and/or obese before pregnancy. They all tend to gain similar amounts of fat. Obese mothers who accumulate fat around their abdomens end up laying it down in the liver and around the pancreas, not only causing problems for themselves (e.g., diabetes of pregnancy) but also making it much more likely for them to have obese or overweight babies. Their children are more likely to develop heart disease and diabetes as adults, and this is even more likely for female children.[16]

Kasia

Kasia's mom worked as a cleaner and took up smoking to avoid eating food. Because her mom smoked during her pregnancy, Kasia was a small baby—6.5 lb. Kasia's mother was employed, so she weaned Kasia onto formula milk as soon as possible so that she could get back to work quickly. Kasia's mom was also convinced that formula milk was better because it cost a lot of money.

Mothers get blamed for a lot for causing obesity in their children. Most of the blame is unjustified and rarely makes it beyond a headline on twitter or in a magazine. Beware the hype. The number of brothers and sisters, the season at birth (i.e., winter), the age of the mother at birth, the number of miscarriages, and when complementary feeding is introduced have all been suggested and disproven.[17]

Conversely, mothers can have an effective role in minimizing the likelihood that their children will grow up with a weight problem. There is good evidence that eating habits start early and stay for life. Breast-feeding reduces the risk of a child becoming overweight by 15%, probably because the amount of breast milk a mother can produce is limited, and so the baby learns about restrained feeding. Breast milk also gives babies a lot of mother protection and developmental guidance. The way it works to prevent babies getting fat is quite specific. Babies and infants who are breastfed can regulate their intakes better. Continuing the restraint into the transition to solids and bottled milk builds up a healthy pathway in a child's brain. Stopping when they are full gets implanted in the brain highways; there is no bottle to empty. When solids are introduced into their diets, they can decrease their milk intake themselves. For bottle-fed babies, solids are often given in addition to milk, and the control of the amount is more in the hands of an anxious parent or caregiver.[18] Putting a child to sleep with a bottle is a recipe for weight disaster.

My mother, like Kasia's mother, smoked during her pregnancies. She told me that the doctors told her that if she smoked, she would have a smaller baby and the delivery would be easier. In fact, the opposite is now true. Smoking during pregnancy leads to bigger babies who gain weight quickly and who are therefore more likely to have weight problems in life. This is probably because mothers who smoke during pregnancy do so to control their appetite and therefore their weight gain. These unhelpful messages about how to regulate appetite pass over to us as babies—even the smoking.[19]

So it was no surprise to me that my most successful weight maintenance strategy in my twenties became smoking. Unfortunately, it was also my most destructive. Without a disruptive weight management plan when I finally managed to stop smoking I put on 60 lb! Now over 20 years later, as a result of even that decade of smoking, my exercise tolerance is 60% of people my age who have never smoked. I am fit but likely never will be fit enough for very vigorous exercise.

It was no wonder I really understood Kasia's story. Her parents were refugees from a war-torn land. They took a boat from one end of the earth to another and wound up in a camp. Compared with where they had come from, the food was plentiful, and her dad started making up for all the years of war starvation. He got fat and stayed that way all the rest of his life. Kasia's parents fed her as if their lives depended on it. A rosy, fat, smart child was what they wanted to see. And they did. Kasia was a fat child and too embarrassed to do any sports or exercise. She was clever and got bored easily, and when she was bored or worried, she ate—and she really liked Western fast food.

At all ages, critical events, such as immigration and migration, can also encourage obesity and overweight. Unhealthy weight gains can come up to 15 years after immigration or migration.[20] Kasia had lifelong problems ahead of her in her new world. However, together we found a way forward to work together on her unhealthy weight. Weight disruption was something she could manage, compared to the disruption of coming to a new land.

> *Our genetics provide the blueprint. Our bodies build the infrastructure. Our lifestyle furnishes it.*

What research into genetics makes increasingly clear is that genetic factors make only a limited contribution to our risk of obesity. If we do carry obesity genes, it is not a given that we will become overweight. As we travel through this book together, it will become clear that disrupting a wide range of strategies and constructing new ones can counteract most effects.

Genes may be procreators, but they are not workers. It is up to many other components both inside and outside our cells—such as hormones, which are involved in how we store and transfer energy within the body—to do the work of living and contribute to weight gain. We now know that the hormones in our gastrointestinal tract, pancreas, and regional fat tissue are regulators of fat entry into our cells.

> *Fat signaling starts in the cell and ascends and descends to all parts of the body.*

Hormones such as ghrelin, leptin, and insulin help to control feeding, and they even also help to motivate our eating behaviors. For example, ghrelin makes us feel hungry, and leptin makes us feel full.[21] They also have an active role in the stomach to regulate our appetite.[22]

It is old thinking that energy balance, feelings of fullness, and body weight are controlled by a highly complex system in our brains. Hormones in our stomachs send signals not only about the volume of what we eat, but also about the caloric content and the quality of food we eat, to our brains to be integrated in many different areas, such as controlling our mood and our sleep patterns. They also have an active role in the stomach to regulate our appetite.[23]

Separating the Truth from the Hype

A lot of research has been conducted into the risk factors for obesity and overweight. In any one year, between 16,000 and 50,000 research articles are published on the causes of obesity. Some relationships have been proven conclusively; others are speculative and yet to be conclusively proven or disproven (this doesn't mean they don't have an effect, just that we can't show enough evidence). Most proven risk factors can be related to genes (parental obesity), events in pregnancy and childhood (smoking during pregnancy, high birth weight, rapid weight gain in infancy, overweight or obesity between 8 and 18 months), and lifestyle factors (poor family eating habits, too little sleep duration and bad timing, too much television).[24,25]

This is where we have to separate the important messages from the hype. Let's look at the research on the effects of television. There is a lot of research showing the harmful effects of TV viewing on children's risk of obesity.[26] More than 80% of all advertisements in children's programming are for fast foods or snacks, and for every hour that children watch TV, they see an estimated 11 food advertisements. Advertising is very effective in getting younger children to request more junk foods from their parents. It is not just in advertisements that food is also unhealthily promoted; it is also in most TV programming and movies. Children see more than 500 food references in programs per week, half of which are for to empty-calorie or high-fat/sugar/salt foods. It seems as though the evidence linking the influence of what children see on television on shaping their food habits is irrefutable.

But is it really?

The picture is not so clear-cut. Advertising also allows parents to make more healthy decisions about what to buy. They are more likely to buy food that is advertised as nutritious, healthy, tasty, and convenient. Most parents recognize the negative influence of advertisements for nutrition-poor foods and try to manage healthy eating habits within their families.

The truth is that watching television doesn't make us put on weight. Sure, the advertisements that blast our senses—especially around meal and snack times—can influence what we want to eat. But it is sitting around for hours in front of a television or sitting around anywhere for that matter, being time we don't spend in calorie-burning activity, and eating in front of the television that sends messages to the brain linking food and inactivity.

> *More than 80% of all advertisements in children's programming are for fast foods.*

It's not all bad news. Overweight viewers who watch public service announcements featuring real people rather than actors had the higher diet, exercise, information seeking and social media word-of-mouth intentions to lose weight.[27] Also, some of the newer interactive video games such as active sports, exercise, and dance videos can be equivalent to moderate-intensity walking.[28]

There is other good news. Depending on where you live, you look at your mobile phone on average between 40 (UK) and 120 (United States) times a day. Health apps on our smartphones may offer a better way to use the visual and auditory technology to control weight. By 2012, there were over 40,000 mobile device applications for health care, and now that number has quadrupled. The most accessed of these health apps are about weight reduction. At the moment, the overall use is low and rarely sustained. In one very large study of a free mobile app for dietary self-monitoring, only 2.58% used it actively. But those who did were healthy eaters or already compliant with strict diets. So if you have a smartphone, put it to use this way in your weight-loss life!

Similar to the TV watching and weight gain claims, not sleeping a fixed number of hours, itself, doesn't spur weight gain. There is no set time that we need to sleep at night. However, hormones that promote healthy growth, not fat deposition, are released after an adequate amount of sleep. That is why sleep is necessary—especially in children. Lack of sleep when we are in our growth phase does indeed increase our risk of obesity. Every hour of sleep that we need but don't get raises the odds of our becoming obese. Sleep helps maintain a healthy balance of the hormones that make you feel hungry or full. When you don't get enough sleep, you have more circulating ghrelin (increasing hunger) and less leptin (creating a sense of fullness).[29] Lack of sleep also results in a higher than normal blood sugar level, which may lead to diabetes.[30] This is true for all age groups, though as we get older and require less sleep, the problem is not as great. Children who are more physically active also sleep longer at night.

I've never been a good sleeper. I find worrying that I am not getting enough sleep usually makes me anxious, and the anxiety triggers a false hunger. In the middle of the night, it is easier to grab a high-calorie, high-carbohydrate, low-nutrition snack than it is to fix something healthy and more weight disruptive. The solution for me has to settle down my anxiety by reminding me to trust that my body and my mind will get the sleep I need. While 6 to 8 hours of sleep is recommended for most adults, there is no fixed amount of sleep absolutely necessary beyond two 90-minute periods of unconsciousness for the brain and adequate muscle relaxation, and no amount of eating will make either happen.

Marcia

Marcia was just turning 12. She entering the most at-risk age group, that is, 12- to 19-year-olds.[31] She also lived in one of the Deep South states where obesity is more acceptable.[32] Obese adolescents are five times more likely to be obese adults than nonobese adolescents. Over half of obese children go on to be obese adolescents, and around 80% of will be obese adults.[33] She was at the crossroad between childhood and adulthood, and although it was a relatively short period in her life, the body changes she was experiencing were powerful signals. All her friends were built like her, with big breasts and butts—the norm in her culture. Marcia also had a large gooseneck and large arms and thighs. None of her friends ate vegetables.[34] They all preferred "diet" or sugar-sweetened soda to plain water.[35] She didn't want to control or confine her foods. She had seen other girls getting depressed and anxious when they started dieting, and she didn't want that to happen to her.[36]

But it wasn't too late for her to change her lifestyle and therefore her weight.

At school, children are subject to a whole new range of environmental risks.[37] Even if parents are diligent about what children eat at home, it is difficult to enforce healthy eating at school. The drive to provide children with healthy packed lunches from home or provide healthier options in school cafeterias doesn't always work.[38] Eighty-five percent of pupils still bring a sweetened soft drink and one nonfruit snack in their packed lunches.

School interventions targeting obesity are successful in the short term because they are imposed in the closed environment of the school, but whether that results in lifelong change is unknown. We now know that strategies that change free time actions are important. That is why programs outside school have shown some promise of sustainability.[39]

Marcia learned that weight management is a lifelong process, that there are no quick fixes. Rapid weight loss is often followed by weight gain. Motivation then wanes, and a new strategy has to be initiated. Modifying our "obesogenic" environment is the first step. Marcia's "ecological niche" was a good place to start. It included the family, the peers, the school, and a closer look at what was happening in the wider society.

Sustainable weight management for Marcia required daily attention to her shame and guilt, a variety of disruptive strategies, and a balance between was subtracted from and what was added to her life. She described it as "like going to the weight management supermarket every day." She would ask herself, "What combination of products should I 'buy' today?" She always had in the back of her mind that focusing on just one intervention for too long would be counterproductive. Gradually she added other strategies, cautious not to overload herself.

She couldn't change her environment as an adolescent, but as a young adult she became more aware of the influences that her surroundings had on her weight. Her neighborhood had a grocery store or fast-food outlet on every corner.[40] She had trained herself to bypass the fast-food outlets and to go to the grocery store on the day the fresh fruit and vegetables were delivered.

The hospital clinic where she saw a dietician was an hour bus ride away—in a bus that didn't have seats to accommodate obese people. She was too scared to use the subway because she couldn't manage the stairs, and there was no private parking at the clinic if she went by car. So she stopped going. Instead, she found diets that could be downloaded as apps on her phone and changed them regularly—depending on what was available and affordable at her local store.

Almost every U.S. adolescent goes online daily; over half do so several times a day; and a quarter do it "almost constantly." The most common site is Facebook (53%), then Instagram (41%), and then Twitter and Pinterest. Over half of all 13- to 32-year-olds have posted a photo on social media of food or drinks that they or someone else was consuming. The most common postings are about unhealthy food and beverage brands.[41] Marcia was one of those adolescents. The effects of the social media onslaught on her took time to be fully understood.

The Future

Understanding how billions of different mechanisms in our bodies operate to moderate fat will require a concerted scientific effort and a new kind of knowledge that integrates what we find with how it works. With such big variations, enormous data sets will have to be developed, and intelligent programming will be required to link the collected data. At the same time, clinical relevance throughout the process will have to be maintained.

This is not the work of one country, or of a single industry, or even of one group of researchers. It will require our own commitment to our future. Big sets of health data are being collected all over the world that could let us look at the factors causing our obesity and compare them with others. To be able to assess the benefits of different treatments for each of us as individuals, both in the short and the long term, would be good shopping—if only we could access and read all the labels easily.

Notes

1. http://www.tandfonline.com/doi/pdf/10.1080/15374416.2016.1152555?need Access=true
2. https://arxiv.org/pdf/1607.01462v1.pdf
3. http://www.tandfonline.com/doi/pdf/10.1080/15374416.2016.1169539?need Access=true
4. Turning WAT into BAT: a review on regulators controlling the browning of white adipocytes. Lo KA, Sun L. *Biosci. Rep.* 2013, 33, 711–719. art:e00065, doi 10.1042/BSR20130046. http://www.bioscirep.org/content/ppbioscirep/33 /5/e00065.full.pdf
5. http://genesdev.cshlp.org/content/27/3/234.full.pdf+html
6. Human brown adipose tissue: regulation and anti-obesity potential. Saito M. *Endocrine Journal* 2014, 61 (5), 409–416. https://www.jstage.jst.go.jp/article/endocrj /61/5/61_EJ13-0527/_pdf
7. Brown fat develops a *brite* future. Klingenspora M, Herzigb S, Pfeifer A. *Obes. Facts* 2012, 5, 890–896. http://www.karger.com/Article/Pdf/346337
8. http://healthyeating.sfgate.com/average-caloric-expenditure-during-olympic -triathlon-12425.html
9. Measuring and Evaluating Body Composition. Esmat T. American College of Sports Medicine. Oct 07, 2016. https://www.acsm.org/public-information/articles /2016/10/07/measuring-and-evaluating-body-composition
10. http://www.mayoclinicproceedings.org/article/S0025-6196(16)30595-X/full text
11. http://physrev.physiology.org/content/physrev/93/1/359.full.pdf
12. http://journals.plos.org/plosone/article?id=10.1371/journal.pone.0058272
13. http://bmcpediatr.biomedcentral.com/articles/10.1186/1471-2431-14-249# Sec1
14. http://www.karger.com/Article/FullText/455952
15. http://www.karger.com/Article/FullText/455952
16. http://press.endocrine.org/doi/full/10.1210/en.2016-1058
17. http://online.liebertpub.com/doi/pdf/10.1089/chi.2015.0055
18. http://online.liebertpub.com/doi/pdfplus/10.1089/chi.2016.0021?src=recsys
19. http://www.arcmedres.com/article/S0188-4409(16)00014-X/fulltext
20. http://link.springer.com/article/10.1186/1471-2458-13-458/fulltext.html

21. http://press.endocrine.org/doi/full/10.1210/en.2016-1058

22. http://press.endocrine.org/doi/full/10.1210/en.2016-1058

23. http://press.endocrine.org/doi/full/10.1210/en.2016-1058

24. http://www.bmj.com/content/330/7504/1357?variant=full-text

25. http://www.ncbi.nlm.nih.gov/books/NBK19935

26. http://download.springer.com/static/pdf/528/art%253A10.1186%252Fs12
889-016-2981-5.pdf?originUrl=http%3A%2F%2Fbmcpublichealth.biomedcen
tral.com%2Farticle%2F10.1186%2Fs12889-016-2981-5&token2=exp=1475510
044~acl=%2Fstatic%2Fpdf%2F528%2Fart%25253A10.1186%25252Fs12889
-016-2981-5.pdf*~hmac=274126a6253e09aa6a082f7ff5b5d9d9679fda7e32d8f7
a63e112d2215bd1080

27. http://www.tandfonline.com/doi/full/10.1080/10810730.2015.1080326
?scroll=top&needAccess=true

28. http://pediatrics.aappublications.org/content/128/1/201.full

29. http://onlinelibrary.wiley.com/doi/10.1038/oby.2007.118/full

30. http://www.nhlbi.nih.gov/health/health-topics/topics/obe/causes

31. http://onlinelibrary.wiley.com/doi/10.1111/mcn.12184/full

32. http://www.sciencedirect.com/science/article/pii/S0749379716302458

33. http://onlinelibrary.wiley.com/doi/10.1111/obr.12334/full

34. http://onlinelibrary.wiley.com/doi/10.1002/oby.21369/abstract

35. http://onlinelibrary.wiley.com/doi/10.1111/cob.12163/full

36. http://journals.plos.org/plosone/article?id=10.1371/journal.pone.0157240

37. http://ajcn.nutrition.org/content/97/6/1178.short

38. https://www.cornwallhealthyschools.org/documents/packed%20lunch%20
toolkit.pdf

39. http://www.nature.com/ijo/journal/v28/n3s/full/0802812a.html

40. http://onlinelibrary.wiley.com/doi/10.1111/j.1467-789X.2010.00769.x/full

41. https://ses.library.usyd.edu.au//bitstream/2123/14967/2/social%20media
%20and%20health%20review.pdf

CHAPTER TWO

We Really Are What We Eat

This chapter explores the latest evidence on diets—how they evolved and the role of commercialization, for example, how trans fats became bad and poly fats became bad and good again; how added sugar is bad, but sugar in genetically sweetened fruits isn't. We will unearth the best evidence and provide some realistic and proven long-term strategies to take the weight off and keep it off—for life.

Dieting and obesity are big business opportunities for both research and commerce. Again, more than 200 scientific articles about obesity are published every day. This avalanche of information can bury any hope of sensible reasoning and make any food or drink healthy or unhealthy—even sugar, salt, and fats. The problem is that we need a lot of the foods that weight reduction diets restrict; for example, we need some of the cholesterol in fat to make our hormones, need some glucose from sugar to feed our brains, and need some salts to keep our blood circulating and our muscles firing.

My Perspective

If you eat nutritious food and pay attention to portions, you don't put on weight. Above all, it is important to make sure that the road to healthy choices is as pleasant as possible and not guilt inducing.

My sustained weight loss required an initial effort to consciously disrupt and change what I ate in order to lose the weight. It took two years to graduate from the basics to advanced understanding. As I became competent at food intervention, and as disruptive rotation became intuitive, I was confident enough to add new strategies to get closer to my ideal weight—always followed by maintenance strategies to keep the weight off.

When we talk about losing weight, we usually focus on dieting and the short-term changes to eating habits that come with diets. However, to lose weight and keep it off, long-term changes need to be made to eating habits. Healthy eating is more than just dieting. To permanently lose weight, a lifetime of healthy habits need to be formed. We need to develop lifelong strategies for weight maintenance after weight loss has been achieved.

Healthy eating is about making healthy food choices, not just limiting quantity. A healthy diet is more than just a feature of a weight-loss program. It is about preventing possible health problems, about changing eating habits for life for a stronger, happier, more active, and therefore better life.

Much of what we eat isn't rich with the ingredients our bodies need.

To maintain a stable weight, our energy output must match energy intake (calories in = calories burned with activities). The energy used by our bodies just to maintain a resting state is called "resting energy expenditure" (REE). REE is calculated differently for males than for females.

For males, REE = 900 + 10 × weight (kg)
For females, REE = 700 + 7 × weight (kg)

Once calculated, the REE must be adjusted for a person's level of physical activity by multiplying × 1.2 for sedentary people, × 1.4 for moderately active people, or × 1.8 for very active people.

What is your current REE?

That final figure is an estimate of the total number of calories we need to stay in energy balance, but we need to understand more to *lose* weight.

For example, a woman weighing 65 kg (143.3 lb) who is moderately active (30 minutes every other day) has an energy requirement of:

$(700 + 7 \times 65) \times 1.4 = 1617$ calories per day

Within a healthy, balanced diet, the current recommendations are that a man, in general, needs around 2,500 calories a day to maintain his weight, and a for a woman, that figure is around 2,000 calories a day.[1] A minimum of 1,200 calories of intake per day for women and 1,500 calories for men should be maintained, unless under careful supervision.

To remain healthy, we need a range of nutrients from several key food groups: proteins, carbohydrates, fats, vitamins, and minerals. The proportions of each group vary according to our genetic makeup and the environment in which we find ourselves. The U.S. Food and Drug Administration (FDA) has a series of recommendations about the optimum amounts of these groups that need to be ingested daily. They recommend that 10–14% of daily intake should be protein, 55% carbohydrate, and a maximum of 30% fat. These recommendations are meant not for weight loss but for weight maintenance in a young and relatively active person.

No one food alone can provide a nutritious diet. A variety of at least 30 different foods over a week are recommended to provide the range of vitamin and mineral nutrients for each of us. Foods that are rich in nutrients rather than high in energy, such as bananas, are healthier for us. A small banana contains seven essential minerals and up to 13 essential vitamin or vitamin subgroups.[2] The lower the energy density (calories) of

At least 30 different foods over a week provide the range of vitamins and minerals we need.

a food eaten, the more likely the body is to "burn" its own fat stores. High-bulk foods, such as pasta in low quantities, may be useful because they help us feel full and discourage our continued eating.

Despite a population that is increasingly obese, many of us have dietary gaps because much of the food we eat is not rich with the types of ingredients our bodies need. For example, the intake of vitamins D and E is below daily requirements for most of us. More than one in three unhealthily weighted people have an inadequate intake of magnesium, calcium, and vitamins A and C. When we are overweight or obese, we tend to have less fiber and potassium in our diets.[3]

Bill and Toni

Bill was obese, and Toni is overweight. Their paths to healthier weight were very different. Bill lost weight more quickly with intensive, low-fat, reducing diets, and it didn't matter if the diet included meal replacements or not.[4] Toni followed the research that suggested she increase her intake of whole grains or total dietary fiber in a major way, and over many years the approach worked.[5]

One benefit of dealing with couples who are both overweight is that you can discuss the issues that relate to couples in a caring way. One of the reasons Bill and Toni came to see me was because Bill was having problems maintaining an erection. They wanted a specific intervention to deal with their sexual problem. They were reassured when I told them it was a common problem, and once I explained to them that all weight-reduction activities improve sexual function—regardless of diet mode—they were relieved and content to try a variety of options.[6]

To remain healthy, we need the range of nutrients from several key food groups: proteins, carbohydrates, fats, vitamins, and minerals, in the proportions recommended by the FDA (previously mentioned).

Protein is essential in our diet to produce amino acids, which are the building blocks of our bodies. Lots of current diets play around with the amount of protein in them. There is no clear justification for any of them. Some promoters of high-protein diets suggest that these diets promote weight loss by increasing our sense of fullness, while others suggest that, even though increased protein leads to muscle development and rather than weight loss, weight is changed from toxic fat to healthy muscle. Either way, proteins can also be used for energy in times of great stress. So-called animal proteins, such as meat, fish, chicken, and eggs are more efficient in delivering protein to our bodies.

There are times during our lives when increasing our protein intake is particularly important: infancy, childhood, adolescence, pregnancy and breast feeding, and as we get old. Meat is the most effective way of getting protein; however, substitutes can be used as long as the amount of protein we eat is sufficient. A variety of regular protein-based foods such as fish, poultry, beans, and meat are good at any age.

Most meats and fish contain some fat, which can add weight. The way the food is cooked can also increase the fat content, for instance, if it is fried or battered. The lowest-fat meats are broiled lean fillet steak, canned ham, boiled chicken, and stewed rabbit. Processed meats such as salami and sausages have the highest fat content. Low-fat seafood include steamed bream, baked cod, oysters, mussels, and prawns.

The next best sources are high-protein vegetables such as runner beans, soya beans, peas, corn, broccoli, pulses (such as lentils), and some cereals. Eggs and dairy products also provide a lot of protein for the ovolactovegetarian diet. However, most egg and dairy products are higher in fat per portion than equivalent lean or low-fat cooked meats and fish. Meat substitutes such as tofu and Quorn, depending on how they are cooked, have relatively low fat content, as do pulses such as lentils.

Our protein intake needs to increase during periods of high growth, such as pregnancy and breast-feeding. Pregnant and breast-feeding women need to double their protein intake with, for example, additional servings of dairy products, making it difficult to assess what is a healthy amount.

Carbohydrates (carbs) are the main source of energy for our bodies. They come in two forms: simple and complex. Simple carbohydrates are energy sources that are more rapidly available, such as sugars. Sugars occur naturally in fruits, honey, malt, milk, and milk products. Many packaged and refined foods contain added sugar, such as candy, cookies, cakes, and pastries, nondiet soda, and syrups in canned fruit. Sugars come in a range of disguises in our foods. The "sugar" we talk about is actually only one of a family of sugars. Its chemical name is sucrose. In drinks and foods, we often find it hidden behind other names: anhydrous dextrose, brown sugar, cane crystals, cane sugar, corn sweetener, corn syrup, corn syrup solids, crystal dextrose, evaporated cane juice, fructose sweetener, fruit juice concentrates, high-fructose corn syrup, honey, liquid fructose, malt syrup, maple syrup, molasses, pancake syrup, raw sugar, sugar, syrup, and white sugar.[7]

The other main types of sugars, some of which we are less able to absorb, include fructose, lactose, and maltose. Fructose is a sugar that is found in mainly derived fruit and vegetables; lactose is the sugar found in milk sugar; and maltose is sugar that comes from grain and grain-based alcohols like whiskey. Sugar has a disproportionate effect on our weight because sugar is very energy efficient. A small amount of sugar can provide a lot of energy—which is readily turned into fat and stored. So even a small amount can push up our weight in a major way. And the effect of sugar can be magnified many times when other conditions, like diabetes or arthritis, are present.

Adding fructose instead of sucrose in place of equal amounts of other carbohydrates (mainly starch or sugar) will not put on any additional weight. Some studies have shown that it will help manage diabetes. However, at high doses, such as >60 g (2.12 oz)/day or >10% of total daily energy, fructose adds to weight gain and the risk of diabetes.[8]

Complex carbohydrates are found in pasta, whole grains, vegetables, and fruit. They are converted to simple carbohydrates to provide energy over a longer period of time. When we are not stressing our bodies, at least half of our daily calorie intake should come from carbohydrates.

Fat is a concentrated source of energy for the body. There are many types of fat, the most common of which are saturated and unsaturated. Saturated fat should be limited to less than 10% of daily calorie intake. It is mainly found in meat and dairy products. Unsaturated fat comes in two types: monounsaturated and polyunsaturated. Monounsaturated fat is found in olive oil. Polyunsaturated fats come from the omega 3 oils found in some fish (mackerel, herring, salmon, and tuna) and nuts and seeds (pumpkin, sesame, and sunflower). Monounsaturated and polyunsaturated fats should make up less than 20% of our daily calorie intake.

Besides their role in shaping hormones in the body (cholesterol), fats are an essential part of our diet. We require some essential fats such as linoleic acid. Other fats are necessary to help essential fat-soluble vitamins A, D, E, and K, to enter our cells.

Fats are essential parts of commercially produced food and drink products. They make food "attractive" in many ways: providing an attractive glossy and translucent appearance, carrying flavors and aromas, making foods melt and feel creamy. In response to the need to decrease fat in food products, companies have been producing substances that mimic fat and replace the fat in a product. Often this comes at a price—sacrificing texture and/or flavor. For both clinical and marketing reasons, partial fat replacement is more common in products.

The types of fats that are deemed bad for our health have been narrowed down over the years. At first it was all saturated fats, and now it is only a particular type of saturated fats, called trans fats, that are problematic. Trans fats are one of the main causes of heart disease. Just a 2% increase in our intake of trans fat can increase our risk of heart and circulation problems by nearly 25%.[9]

While trans fats have been banned and are being phased out by mid-2018 in the U.S. food supply, it is difficult to remove them from processed foods because they are an important way of extending the shelf life of these products. The major products that still have trans fat at this writing are crackers, cookies, cakes, frozen pies and other baked goods, snack foods (such as some microwave popcorn), margarines, coffee creamers, refrigerated dough products, and ready-to-use frostings.

Lucie

Lucie was 40 years old and weighed 205 kg (450 lb) when she decided to have bariatric surgery. She suffered from high blood pressure and diabetes, both of which went away when her BMI returned to 25. It was explained to her that she had to stay on nutritional supplements, such as multivitamins and minerals with extra doses of calcium and vitamin D, for the rest of her life. She moved to a new home once she was stable because she couldn't stand the way people looked at her and commented about her weight loss. She wanted to start somewhere new as a "thin person."

Six years later, she returned to her original home. She had broken her arm on an icy street and decided to return to the city she knew. Her arm didn't heal very well, and she had an ongoing infection. She also said she had problems with a sore tongue, and her hair was getting thin. She noticed she was very pale, but she thought that was because she didn't get out in the sun very much. These were all symptoms of micronutrient deficiency. She said she had stopped "worrying" about taking supplements once her weight had stabilized.

When we adopt restrictive diets or remove part of our capacity to absorb micronutrients, quite often we become deficient in essential nutrients, especially if they occur only in small amounts in even a normal diet. These micronutrients are mainly vitamins and minerals. For example, vitamin A is carried into the body only in fat, and very low-fat diets can cause vitamin A deficiency. Vitamin A plays an important role in many functions of our bodies: vision, bone growth, immune system, reproduction, and cell growth. It also maintains the surface linings of the eye, the respiratory, urinary, and intestinal tracts. Whole eggs, whole milk, and liver are among the few foods that naturally contain vitamin A. Vitamin A is present in the fat portion of whole milk and is not found in fat-free milk. If you are using fat-free milk in a low-fat diet, it is important to check that the milk you are using has added vitamin A.

Other fat-soluble vitamins that we need to watch out for if we are on a low-fat diet are vitamins D and E. The major function of vitamin D is to maintain normal blood levels of calcium and phosphorus, which are responsible for strong bones and muscle contractions. Vitamin D is found in food but also can be made in the body after exposure to ultraviolet rays from the sun. Fortified foods, such as milk and cereal, are the major dietary sources of vitamin D. Lucy had a severe vitamin D deficiency, which caused her bones to be brittle and break with the smallest provocation.

Vitamin E is a powerful antioxidant that acts to protect our cells against the effects of free radicals, which are potentially damaging by-products of our body's metabolism. It is also involved in keep a healthy immune, or protective, system. Lucie's ongoing infection on her arm was a result of an impaired immune system. Vegetable oils, nuts, green leafy vegetables, and fortified cereals are the main dietary sources of vitamin E.

All the other important vitamins are water soluble and so don't require fat to accompany them into our bodies. However, because they are in small quantities in the food we eat, we still can experience shortages if we stay on too restrictive a diet or as a result of decreased absorption after bariatric surgery.

Vitamin B is mainly found in meat, fish, and poultry. Those of us who chose a diet that is ovolactovegetarian, vegetarian, or vegan need to make sure we get enough vitamin B through sources such as cereals and beans. It is needed to make proteins and blood cells and also helps our nervous and immune systems work properly. Vitamin B is very useful in assisting weight loss when we are on a low-calorie diet because a particular type of vitamin B—B6—helps to convert our carbohydrate to glucose in order to maintain normal blood sugar levels and to feed our brains when we are reducing our food intake.

Folate and folic acid accompany vitamin B and are necessary for the production and maintenance of new cells, which is especially important during periods of rapid cell division and growth, such as infancy and pregnancy. Leafy greens such as spinach, turnip greens, dry beans and peas, fortified cereals and grain products, and some fruits and vegetables are rich food sources of folate. Folic acid as tablets are often given to pregnant women.

Vitamin C helps our bodies absorb iron and to make antioxidants. It is also important in hormone production and healthy cell function. Vitamin C is found mainly in citrus fruits, green vegetables (especially broccoli), tomatoes, and potatoes.

Restrictive diets can also have a deleterious effect on the essential salts and minerals we require for functioning. Iron is an essential mineral and an important backbone of our red blood cells. Lucie's paleness and her ongoing infection were a result of too little iron in her diet to make red blood cells. Almost two-thirds of the iron in the body is found in hemoglobin, the protein in red blood cells that carries oxygen to our tissues. We store about 15% of the iron we ingest for future needs, and this store is mobilized when our dietary intake is inadequate, such as when we are on diets low in iron or when we have other problems such as heavy menstrual bleeding. There are two forms of dietary iron: heme and nonheme. Iron in meat, fish, and poultry is found in a chemical structure known as heme. Heme iron is absorbed very efficiently by the body. Iron in plants such as lentils and beans is arranged in a different chemical structure called nonheme. Nonheme iron is not as easily absorbed as heme iron. Flours, cereals, and grain products that are enriched or fortified with iron are good dietary sources of nonheme iron. So vegetarians or vegans have to work much harder on their diets to make sure they get enough iron—especially when menstruating.

Magnesium is a mineral needed by every cell of our body. It helps to maintain our normal muscle and nerve function, to keep our heart rhythm steady, and to make our bones strong. It is also involved in energy metabolism and protein synthesis. Green vegetables such as spinach provide magnesium. Nuts, seeds, and some whole grains are also good sources of magnesium.

Selenium is a mineral involved in protecting our cells. It works with antioxidant enzymes to control free radical damage to cells and can reduce the impact of chronic diseases like arthritis. Selenium is also essential for the normal functioning of the immune system and thyroid gland. Thyroid problems are more common in those of us who have had bariatric surgery. Plants are the major dietary source of selenium. The amount of selenium in soil, which varies by region, determines the amount of selenium in the plants that are grown in a given region. Selenium also can be found in some meats and seafood. Some nuts, in particular Brazil nuts and walnuts, are also very good sources of selenium.

Zinc is an essential mineral that is found in almost every cell in the body. It is important for a healthy immune system, for healing cuts and wounds, and for maintaining our senses of taste and smell. Lucie was clearly suffering from zinc deficiency. Zinc also supports normal growth and development during pregnancy, childhood, and adolescence. Meat and poultry provide the majority of zinc in the diet. Other food sources include beans, nuts, and dairy products. Oysters contain the most zinc by weight, but beef is a more common source. Specific dietary proteins called phytates, which are found in whole grain cereals and unleavened bread, may significantly decrease our absorption of zinc.

Calories and Cutting Them

A calorie is a measure of body energy. It can be used to describe what we put into our bodies, such as food, or what we use up, such as in exercise. Here are the calorific values of the three main components of the food we eat:

1 g of carbohydrates contains 4 calories (1 oz = 114 calories)

1 g of protein contains 4 calories (1 oz = 114 calories)

1 g of fat contains 9 calories. (1 oz = 255 calories)

In many regions, including the European Union, Australia, and New Zealand, it has become standard practice to include energy data in food labels in joules (J, or kilojoules, kj) instead of kilocalories (calories).

1 J = 0.239005736 of a calorie, or 1 calorie = 4.18 J

Almost every packaged food today features calorie counts in its label. These can be very useful in comparing products but are not that useful in assessing what we should eat. I have a couple of pet nutrients that I always check—fat content and calories. Fat content is sometimes hard to work out because some labels measure it as a percentage (the maximum recommended percentage is 10%), while other labels measure the fat content in grams or ounces (30 g, or 1oz, is the recommended daily maximum). Also, when labels designate that the product is "fat free" or "lite," it usually means that more sugar or artificial sweetener has been added to improve the taste in the absence of fat.

The best form of defense against being unhealthy is vigilance. Many foods today carry labels and advertising that make you think they are healthier, lower fat, or lower sugar than others. It is best to read the labels to check. The fat content of food matters more to us when we are obese or overweight. Adding three tablespoons of olive oil to our meal is the same as adding three scoops of ice cream.[10]

The top six dangerously fat-rich food groups are (1) butter, oils, lard, animal fat, meat drippings; (2) fatty cuts of meats; (3) margarine, mayonnaise, salad dressings; (4) nuts, seeds, seed kernels; (5) peanut butter, chocolates, candies, potato chips, cookies, trail mix; and (6) cheese. The top six dangerously sugar-rich foods are (1) sugar, honey; (2) soft drinks (not diet drinks); (3) candy; (4) jelly; (5) cakes, puddings, biscuits, pastries; and (6) ice cream.

How many calories we extract from food depends not only on what we eat but also on how we prepare our food, which bacteria are in our gut, and how much energy we use to digest different foods.[11] Current calorie counts do not consider any of these factors. Our digestion is so intricate and changeable that even if we try to improve calorie counts on labels, we will likely never make them perfectly accurate. The best strategy is to continually check which foods are the most energy efficient for us individually. What might work for our partners or children may not work for us. This can make mealtimes complex and up for some negotiation. Our body systems are very amenable to change, so diets are always very helpful in the beginning of a weight-loss program. However, our bodies are also very good at adapting to what they are used to. The best way to deal with this is to be flexible and change your diets when you plateau or gain.

Bassey

Bassey is obese and over 6′ tall. He has lost up to 63 lb (28.5 kg) several times but has put it back on again within the space of a year. When he loses it, he can exercise and frequently completes 10-km (6-mile) runs. After a month or so, when his weight loss begins to plateau, he gets bored and less strict, and he often starts to consume extra food. Sometimes, like Bassey, we get trapped in a cycle of rapidly losing and regaining weight. This is called "yo-yo dieting." At the outset of dieting, most people are enthusiastic to lose weight and take great care to stick to the diet. After a week or a month or so, when weight loss begins to plateau, people become bored and less strict, and they often consume extra food. Such yo-yo dieting can lead to a slower metabolic rate and impede long-term weight loss.

Bassey and his partner came around for dinner. They had told me beforehand that they were on diets and so weren't drinking alcohol. I made a low-fat seafood bisque with rice. Bassey put a small amount of food on his plate and then asked me if there was any bread. I said no. He looked disappointed. As an experiment to test their diet resolve, I offered them some leftover fruitcake for dessert. I put three medium-sized pieces on a sharing plate. Bassey cut one piece into little sections, and we all took one of the small pieces. By the time they left, Bassey had eaten the remaining two pieces.

Bassey asked me how the book was going and about its theme. I told him it explains weight loss and how weight maintenance is a lifelong activity. Relapses are common but need to be learned from and managed. He smiled, a little embarrassed. He then asked me what I thought the book might do for him. The most important thing for him was to stop using yo-yo dieting as his weight management activity. He needed to try other things. I suggested he try an elimination technique.

I made him list his top 10 favorite foods in descending order of preference: fruit; fruit cake; his partner's chocolate cake (she was at the table looking lovingly at him at the time); and vegetables. Then he stopped. I said what about scones and cream and buttered toast? I had seen him devour both when we met for a holiday. He went away and sent me more of the list on Facebook: buttered bread, all cakes, and watermelon.

Realistically, we weren't going to get to number 10—but that wasn't important. What I was aiming to do was to help him identify something he liked but that he could also eliminate forever. A longer list just gave him more choices.

I first tried this exercise in my twenties, when I told myself that I really didn't like chocolate. It was number 10 on my list. I have the occasional chocolate now, but usually it is because someone is trying to prove that it is the ultimate chocolate that will convince me that I like chocolate. I rarely finish a piece. My mind and body don't relate to chocolate anymore.

Over time, with each elimination success, we can stop controlling what we eat and enjoy what we like that is healthy. My favorite foods change frequently because I want to keep disrupting what my body likes. My current top likes are bread, which I have reduced to only three types that I like enough to eat (German rye, French-style baguette, or sourdough); mayonnaise, but only a Japanese brand that is hard to find; hummus, but only low fat without garlic, which is also hard to find; chili, which I use with nearly every lunch or dinner to stimulate my bowels and speed elimination; and vegetables with high fluid content, which can be excreted quite quickly (e.g., lettuce and celery).

Our Eating Patterns

When our bodies feel full, we should stop eating because we don't feel hungry anymore. This not always the case. A lot of factors influence how we get this feeling of fullness to switch on, for example, how much energy is in the food, what it is made from, what it looks, smells, and tastes like.[12] It is a delicate balance, though, between the type of food we eat and how much of it we eat. Dairy products, for example, can make us feel full, but they also add weight and increase bad cholesterol if taken in large amounts.[13] Capsaicin, which is the major ingredient in chili peppers, can make us feel full and reduce our intake. It is my favorite filler when I have to eat out. I used to carry a jar with me. You have to get used to it, though, and gradually build up your tolerance because initially it can cause pain, burning sensation, nausea, and bloating.[14]

Of course, we don't always stop eating when we start to feel full and quite often snack when we are not hungry. The idea that snacking isn't bad has now been disproven. It really comes down to what we chose to snack on and how much. If you chose foods high in protein, fiber, and whole grains (e.g., nuts, yogurt, prunes, and popcorn), they can make you feel full when snacking.[15] On the other hand, drinking a can of soda every day produces a weight gain of 15 lb (6.8 kg) per year. Nearly 40% of children's caloric intake comes from solid fat and added sugars, and soda or fruit drinks provide nearly 10% of their total calories.[16]

The speed at which we eat is important only if we eat too quickly, thereby not allowing our brain to tell us we are full. Unfortunately, eating more slowly, though it might stop excess intake, hasn't been shown to be helpful in losing weight.[17]

No Diet Is a Magic Bullet for All

There is no magic diet that is better than any other in helping people lose weight. Most people first chose a diet that suits their dietary preferences and lifestyle.[18] Traditionally, calorie-controlled diets have been used to produce rapid weight loss. To use a calorie-controlled diet successfully, we must overcome the initial decrease in energy that accompanies a lower-calorie intake.

Erica weighed herself every other day and skipped breakfast if she hadn't lost weight. But when she did eat breakfast, and it was high in calories and low in nutrients. She often took up diets that were based on one particular type of food, such as high-fiber diets, but she found if she stayed on that diet too long, she had a lot of gas and spent too much time in the bathroom. When she went on a dairy-free diet, the lack of sufficient protein and calcium affected her nails.

Erica had unrealistic expectations of diets. Like many of us, she had a common belief about weight loss. She believed that the promises of losses in excess of 1.1 to 2.2 lb per week would go on for as long as she was on the diet. In reality, the early losses were just fluid loss.

Several well-known diets have proven benefits in weight loss. They usually fall into four categories: low-carbohydrate diets, such as Atkins and South Beach; low-fat, such as Ornish and modified Atkins; higher unsaturated fat, such as Mediterranean; and low glycemic index, such as Pritikin. The Atkins diet is based on the concept that by limiting carbohydrate intake, we force our bodies to stop storing carbohydrates and to have only enough carbs to burn in our daily activities. Low-carbohydrate diets, like the Atkins diet, are typically are high in protein and fat. High protein in the diet is supposed to make us feel full, so we stop eating. The diet is divided into three phases: (1) induction: where we eat less than 20 g (0.71 oz) of carbs per day for 2 weeks; (2) then, for ongoing weight loss, we limit carb intake to 25–45 g (0.88–1.59 oz) per day; (3) in the premaintenance phase, carbs go up to typically 30–60 g (1.06–2.12 oz) per day and finally, in the maintenance phase, carbs are typically 40–100 g (1.41–3.53 oz) per day. Since its publication, this diet has gone through many versions, for example, modified (low fat) and eco(vegetarian).

Restricting carbs too much at the onset will work in the short term as a disruption, but the stress to our bodies of severely restricting carbs for too long will switch on our adaptive mechanisms and make us take more nutrients out of the food we eat. This energy efficiency will put a halt to our weight loss.

Restrictive diets last for only short periods of time before our minds and bodies get wise and find ways of overcoming our strategies.

A spin-off from the Atkins diet is the South Beach diet. The idea behind this diet is that there are two types of carbs—good and bad. We get addicted to bad carbs and should eat only good ones (i.e., low-carb foods like low-carb vegetables). This adaptation is a quite sensible disruption, but for maintenance we really need to graduate to a low-carb diet, and doing so immediately after a low-carb diet is unlikely to work because our bodies are already used to extracting as many carbs as possible from what we eat. This diet should be tried at another time.

A better strategy is to switch to a diet that operates on another concept, such as moderating our fat intake rather than our carbohydrate intake. Low-fat diets, like the Ornish diet, restrict calories from fat to 10–20% of the total diet—about 30 g (1.06 oz) a day. Some fat is essential to ingest important nutrients (as discussed in the previous chapter), but it should be limited.

These diets provide us fewer calories in higher portions, which is also supposed to make us feel full and are best suited for those of us who have weight problems without any associated heart problems.

Rather than restricting the amount of fat we eat, other diets encourage fat intake. Mediterranean-type diets encourage a higher intake of healthy fats such as olive oil, nuts, and fish rather than unhealthy fats (e.g., red meat and butter). These diets are based on the observation that people living around the Mediterranean have less heart disease, so these diets best fit when our weight problems are accompanied by heart problems.

It is not surprising that research is inconclusive as to whether a low-carbohydrate or a low-fat diet is more effective for weight loss. Both work—but only in the short to medium term. Recent medical attention has focused on which of these diets is better for cardiovascular health. Diets high in polyunsaturated (8% of the diet) and monounsaturated fats (17%) raise HDL cholesterol (the healthier carrier of cholesterol). Triglyceride (another fat that can be harmful in excess) was higher in high-carbohydrate diets.[19]

When diabetes or the way we metabolize sugar is the problem, a diet that is low in sugar is best, for example the Pritikin diet. These diets are based on the glycemic index, which was developed in 1981 to help diabetics rank foods according to their immediate effects on blood sugar levels. The glycemic index (GI) is a measure of the relative time it takes for carbohydrate to be converted into energy-giving glucose. The longer the time is, the lower the glycemic index and the better the control of the body's access to glucose. Low-GI foods include whole grain breads, some cereals, pasta, and legumes (baked beans and lentils), fruits, and dairy products like milk and yogurt. The Pritikin diet is based on the concept that if we eat a diet that is high in bulk and fiber—both of which have low carbs—we will feel full and not want to eat anymore and at the same time lose weight. Pritikin meals should contain: 50–75% carbohydrate calories, relatively less meat, fish, fats, and oils and more grains, cereals, breads, fruits, vegetables.

And, every so often, a new fad diet makes it into Twitter or the glossy magazines. Like most diets, they all can achieve a similar weight loss in the short term. The problem is that the explanation of these diets is quite often a flawed piece of logic. Take the Paleolithic (Paleo) diet. It arises from an unsupported assertion that human evolution stopped at the Stone Age and that our genes can't cope with our modern diet and lifestyle. Only foods that were available to hunter–gatherer groups should be eaten: Meat, fruit, and vegetables are acceptable, but grains and dairy products are not. Over 24 months, there is generally no difference in weight reduction between this diet and more established diets, such as the Mediterranean diet. However, the Paleo diet is approximately 10% more expensive than an ordinary diet of similar nutritional value, and the lack of dairy products poses a problem with ensuring enough calcium intake for healthy bones.[20]

Irrespective of the diet we chose, the amount we eat is still most critical. Most of us can't estimate portion sizes very well and so inaccurately estimate our calorie intake. This is an even bigger problem if we rely on prepared foods. Portion sizes of ready-made foods have increased by 200 to 500% in recent years.[21]

In the long run, one weight-loss program is rarely enough for us to maintain our weight loss. All programs are effective in the short term, so the best strategy is to rotate them over a number of years with some breaks in between to see how successful we are without a program. So, when choosing a program, it is best to first recall what programs worked for us before, what we liked, what we didn't like, what made us stop, and so on.[22]

Here are some tips to aid success:

1. Review the package before buying into a diet.

    a. Does it have a specific meal plan or ask you to keep food records? If you have done that before, did you have some success?

    b. If you tried this type of program, why are you considering it again? Do you feel hopeful that it can work again? There is no value in choosing a type of program that didn't work before or that didn't help you develop long-term strategies to keep your weight manageable.

    c. If you haven't tried this type of program, why are you considering it now? Can you make that fit in with your current lifestyle?

2. Do you have to buy special meals or supplements?

    a. Producers are aware of offering variety, but can you make changes based on your likes, dislikes, food allergies, or cultural and religious restrictions?

3. What does the total program cost? Are there hidden extras, such as membership fees, fees for extra payments for special foods, meal replacements, supplements, or other products? Is it affordable?

4. How will you feel for months on end eating differently from the rest of the family? Will you still be okay to prepare their meals, if you do, without snacking on them?

5. Does the program have a plan for problem times like social or holiday eating, changes to your work schedules, or if you become ill or lose motivation?

6. Does the product or program carry any risks? Could the program hurt you? Could the suggested drugs or supplements harm your health?

7. What results do other people in the program typically have? Can you talk to someone who was roughly like you? Do you have written information on these results?

With regular practice, we can get used to estimating portion sizes and calorie or fat counts. There are commercial tools to help us. There are plates with markings for carbohydrates, proteins, cheese, sauce, and vegetables, as well as cereal bowls with markings for different-calorie cereals. As we can expect, using these utensils does result in a significant long-term change in weight, but they are also a useful short-term disruption. Limiting large portions by using presized diet foods promotes initial weight loss, but it is not sustainable in the longer term.[23] That is why disrupting our patterns is the best strategy. Varying our portion sizes can help maintain the momentum until we are comfortable with the portion sizes that work to keep us in a healthy weight range. For example, one month we might decide to have larger breakfasts and smaller dinners, perhaps by respectively increasing and decreasing the protein in each of those meals. The next month we can reverse that. Another strategy is to replace foods temporarily; for example, "Swap it, don't stop it."[24]

Try training yourself. Prepare the same meal once a week for a month. Take a photo of each of the meals and compare the four photos at the end of the month. Were the portion sizes all the same? Prepare an album and a yearly calendar reminder to do it again.

Weight-Loss Programs

Despite years of well conducted research, there is no clear answer as to which formal weight-loss program is best. All diets seem to achieve weight loss or other benefits such as lowered cholesterol, blood sugar, or blood pressure in the short term—some even up to several months. So it is not surprising that the guidelines from the American Heart Association, American

College of Cardiology, and The Obesity Society advise doctors to consider referring patients to any commercial programs with proven effects. Commercially available weight-loss programs are $2.5 billion industry. Ten to 15% of patients who need to lose weight for medical reasons are using commercial programs. Weight Watchers (45%), Nutrisystem (14%), and Jenny Craig (13%) have the largest market shares. In general, weight-loss differences between programs are small.

It is difficult to compare programs when not all of them are studied the same way or for the same length of time. Some programs have been compared with doing nothing. For example, Weight Watchers achieved 2.5–5.9% greater weight loss, whereas Nutrisystem had a 6.7% greater loss when compared with doing nothing, but by three months there were no differences between the two programs.[25] Other programs have been compared against each other; for example, Curves participants lost 1.8 kg (4 lb) more than Weight Watchers participants at three months.

Another way of comparing programs was to see their effect on the medical conditions that accompany obesity, such as the program's ability to help control our blood pressure. For example, Atkins has been compared with SlimFast to show differences in blood pressure, not weight. SlimFast participants had an average of 4.5 mmHg lower systolic blood pressure after six months of follow-up but no difference in diastolic blood pressure, and this finding is difficult for even me as a clinician to understand what it means! At 12 months, Weight Watchers showed little change in blood pressure or lipid outcomes, as compared with doing nothing or participating in health education.

Some studies look at adding counseling to the diet. Weight Watchers and Jenny Craig achieve significantly greater weight losses at one year, compared to people getting nothing or education or counseling. At 12 months, Atkins participants had a better lipid profile than people just going to counseling.[26] Other programs like Nutrisystem, Medifast, and the Biggest Loser Club were also studied, but they did not have any yearlong studies to compare.[27]

We need to practice disruptive dieting. We have to change our diets often so that our bodies don't get used to one way of eating . . . and we must do so for a long period of time.

Up to now, research has shown only small differences between programs and only in the short term. The results are also presented as group findings, so it is difficult to understand what is really happening to each individual.

Unfortunately, very few commercial programs have information on longer-term sustained weight loss. Obesity is a chronic problem, and changes in weight need to be maintained over decades, not months or years. Even when a program shows a sustained weight loss, it is small; for example, both low-fat and low-carbohydrate diets show an average of 1.8 kg (4 lb) loss after two years.[28]

Some longer-term research on very-low-calorie (<800 kcal/day) or low-energy liquid-formula (>800 kcal/day) diets shows promise. These portion-controlled, vitamin- and mineral-fortified, prepackaged diets contain a known energy and nutrition content, usually in the form of a bar or shake. One of the best known is Medifast. These diets can help us achieve weight loss of greater than 15–20%,[29] and such rapid weight loss can be very motivating. By using liquid shakes and meal bars to replace two meals and two snacks a day, we can end up with a weight loss of 7.1 kg (15.7 lb) in three months. If the replacement is continued as one meal and one snack a day, our loss can go up to 10.4 kg (22.9 lb) by 27 months.[30] The initial loss, when combined with a behavioral program, is nearly 4 kg (8.82 lb) after one year. But by two years, the loss was reduced to less than 1.5 kg (3.31 lb). Five percent of this loss can be maintained for four years.[31]

However, these diets are not sustainable for everyone, and weight loss is variable. They are quite often used in preparation for bariatric surgery because they reduce our intake of food so much that our liver shrinks, and this makes the surgery easier. This virtual starvation can cause many medical problems (e.g., to our bones in the form of osteoporosis), so it is no wonder that one in five people on one of these diets stops before the full course.

Fasting

Not eating, of course, is the ultimate weight-loss strategy: but does it really work? And is it healthy? In many religions, some version of fasting is attached to enhance spiritual practice, but there have been very few studies looking at regular fasting as a sustainable weight-loss strategy. Intermittent fasting comes in many forms—alternate day fasting, periodic fasting, or intermittent energy restriction. Usually this kind of diet involves intermixing normal daily diet with a short period of severe calorie restriction or fasting. Weekly fasting periods differ: Some people use intermittent calorie restriction of between two and four days per week; others have two and five days fasting per week. A *fast day* is one where there is either no energy intake (neither food nor drink) or where the intake is reduced. Fast days alternate with "feast" days, on which people can eat as much as they like. Another popular diet, is the five- and-two regime, which is five feast days followed by two fast days.

Weight losses between the fasting regimens vary over the first six months, depending on the diet, but, as with all diet programs, plateaus are reached. For example, the week-on/ week-off strategy results in monthly losses in the first three months of 10.7 kg (23.6 lb), 6.5 kg (14.3 lb), and 8.4 kg (18.5 lb) but results in a final reduction of only 2.1 kg (4.63 lb) in body weight at six months.[32] The rapid weight loss in the beginning is usually the result of water loss rather than fat loss (see Chapter 3). The resulting tiredness, dizziness, and low energy levels cause about one in five people to stop these diets even before they get bored or reach a plateau.[33]

> *Most diets are capable of producing short-term changes, and these changes have to be built upon, not just lost and replaced.*

Crash diets cause all body systems to crash. They cause a loss of muscle equal to the amount of fat lost. When we stop them, to get our levels of energy back, we usually regain both fat and muscle. In addition to being an ineffective form of sustained weight loss, crash diets can cause significant health problems. For example, fasting increases the cholesterol content of bile, which in turn can cause inflammation of the gallbladder (cholecystitis). Gallstones and gallbladder disease are also known complications of extreme diets. Between 10 and 20% of people who have rapid weight reduction using a very low-calorie diet develop gallstones.

That is why we need to practice disruptive dieting. We have to change our diets often so that our bodies don't get used to one way of eating. Fortunately, so many diets are around with new ones coming out every week that we can be disruptive for the five to ten years we might need to get a place where disruption is no longer necessary.

> *Fortunately, there are so many diets around that we can be disruptive for the five to ten years that we need to firmly establish a routine of healthy eating.*

Fluids

When dieting is mentioned, people always think about food. But what we drink is also a significant part of our energy intake. It is very important to maintain our daily water intake; most of our bodies are made up of fluids. We should aim to consume between 1.5 and 2 L (50–70 fluid oz) of water every day (6–8 standard drinks/glasses). Healthy drinking also involves reviewing the amount and types of other liquids that we consume. Alcohol contains a lot of sugar, and yet it is not clear whether drinking alcohol leads to obesity. Light to moderate drinkers (up to 30 g/day or three standard drinks/glasses) are less likely to gain weight than nondrinkers or heavy drinkers. Heavy intake, however, can put on weight. A beer intake of 500 mL/day (two standard drinks or glasses) results in abdominal obesity in men.[34]

By contrast, increasing sugar-sweetened beverage or fruit juice intake causes greater weight. Women who increase their daily intake of water, coffee (without added sugar), or a diet beverage by one serving lose more weight over a four-year period.[35]

The Diet Wars—Which Is Winning?

None—in the long term. No diet has yet been shown as easier to stick with than any other in the long run.[36] Any diet has rules about what a person can and can't eat. That is why a new strategy such as disruption is important because we can change the rules when the old ones stop working. Most diets are capable of producing short-term changes, and these changes have to be built upon, not just lost and replaced. Some diets can lead to slightly better results than others. However, that really doesn't matter. Obesity is a chronic condition, and so it is what can be maintained in the long term that really matters. A disruptive diet plan for clinical weight management needs to be established over timescales of years to decades. Table 2.1 summarizes what we know about the food and drink we ingest and how useful it is in helping us disrupt our weight for life.[37]

Why Do We Fail to Lose Weight on Diets?

Our bodies are very good at controlling our energy balance. We are extremely sensitive to negative energy balance (less calories) but comparatively tolerant of positive energy balance (more calories than we need). This is thought to be a genetic leftover of humans from the past, when food supplies were scarce or unpredictable. Powerful brain systems in place to assure that we don't die of starvation will override other messages that regulate eating and douse our drive to consume energy-dense, high-sugar, and high-fat foods beyond what we need. So it is a mixture of environment and genetic makeup that controls our hunger (the biggest reason for dietary failure) and our food choices.[38]

Table 2.1   The Dietary Courtroom

The Defendant	Unanimous Decision	Majority Decision	Hung Jury	Judges Call
Fruits, nonstarchy vegetables, nuts, seeds, legumes, yogurt	Beneficial			
Dietary fiber, potassium	Beneficial			
Moderate alcohol use	Beneficial			
Mediterranean-style diet	Beneficial			
Partially hydrogenated vegetable oils, processed meats	Harmful			
High sodium	Harmful			
Sugar-sweetened beverages, foods rich in refined grains, starches, added sugars	Harmful			
Greater than moderate alcohol use	Harmful			
Total fat	Little effect			
Seafood, whole grains		Beneficial		
Certain vegetable oils (e.g., soybean, canola, extra virgin olive)		Beneficial		
n-3 and n-6 polyunsaturated fats, plant-derived monounsaturated fats		Beneficial		
Moderate salt		Harmful		
White potatoes		Harmful		
High glycemic index		Harmful		
Total carbohydrate		Little effect		
Antioxidants, vitamins, calcium		Little effect		
Cheese, low-fat milk			Beneficial	
Certain vegetable oils (e.g., corn, sunflower, safflower)			Beneficial	

(continued)

Table 2.1   (*continued*)

The Defendant	Unanimous Decision	Majority Decision	Hung Jury	Judges Call
Coffee, tea, cocoa			Beneficial	
Vitamin D, magnesium			Beneficial	
Saturated fats, dietary cholesterol			Harmful	
Unprocessed red meats, eggs, butter			Harmful	
Poultry			Little effect	
100% fruit juice			Little effect	
Total protein, specific amino acids			Little effect	
Noncaloric sweeteners			Little effect	
Whole-fat milk				Beneficial/ Harmful
Starchy vegetables other than potatoes				Beneficial
Coconut oil				Beneficial
Concepts of local, organic, farmed/wild, grass fed				Little effect
Genetic modification				Little effect

For chronic dieters or restrained eaters, another factor comes into play—the conflict between enjoyment and weight control. As chronic dieters, we often fail in food-rich environments because we are surrounded by food sensations that are linked to the pleasure of eating.[39] However, we all can become restrained eaters over time. Through a continuous process of disruption over several years, we can draw on our past success in exerting self-control and link high-calorie food with weight control thoughts.

Healthy Shopping

Healthy eating often begins with shopping. There are many guides to help us buy wisely. Some health centers run healthy shopping tours, but remember that just going to an organic or healthy supermarket is not a way to lose weight. We have to buy the healthy options like fruit and vegetables![40]

Often we know the appropriate product choice, but another product just "slips" into the cart. To prepare for those occasions or when there is some doubt about what to choose, here are a few tips. Make a list before shopping to avoid buying something unhealthy on impulse, and stick to the list. You might try to plan a nonfood goodie to buy, instead of empty-calorie foods. When shopping, be wary of sales (which are most often junk food), and be wary even if a healthy food is on sale; it may be close to its "use by" date, so inspire an I-need-to-eat-it-fast feeling.

It is less tempting to shop after you have eaten, as people generally buy more—and are subject to impulse buys—when they are hungry. I try go when I am feeling relaxed and not anxious. It helps me make reasonable choices. I try to go to supermarkets I know and avoid the "unhealthy" aisles, but if I am in a new store, I can usually figure out where the fattening food is kept—near the front and at the registers! That doesn't mean I always avoid those aisles, I just start in the low-fat, low-calorie aisles, such as the fruit and vegetables aisles.

Substituting foods is a very useful disruptive shopping strategy. When looking at previous lists, we can see the patterns we fall into. Some low-fat substitutions include jellies instead of chocolate and dried fruit instead of nuts. Creating a disruptive shopping plan can help break that cycle. Table 2.2 presents an example of one I have used in the past to disrupt my fat intake.

> *Vigilance about healthy eating is as important as sleep.*

Reading Food Labels

Most products now also display nutrition information, which lists the amount of energy, protein, fat, carbohydrate, dietary fiber, and the other nutritional components of products. The ingredients listed on the label appear in order of quantity in the product, from highest amount to the lowest—not necessarily in their energy, calorie, or fat value. The term "serving size" relates to the average serving of a product. When comparing products, check that the serving sizes of both are equal before comparing the nutritional content. Sometimes the recommended serving size is much smaller than we would use, and so the product looks healthier. Yet this amount may not relate to what we are used to as a serving size; for example, a small tub of yogurt has two servings per pack. If you use the whole

Table 2.2 My Disruptive Shopping Plan

	My "Usual" Purchases		My Disruptive Choices		
Food Item	Serving Size	Fat/ Serving Size	Alternative Food Item	Serving Size	Fat/ Serving Size
Butter/ margarine	1 T	16 g	Honey/nonfat spread	1 T	0 g
Chicken	100 g breast roasted with skin	13 g	Tuna in brine (not yellow fin)	100 g	1 g
Cottage cheese	Half cup	6 g	Low-fat processed cheese slices	1 slice	3.5 g
Croissant	1 large, plain	17 g	Wholemeal bread	1 slice	1 g
Ice cream, regular, vanilla	1 regular scoop	5 g	Oranges and strawberries	1 c	0 g
Chocolate bar	60 g	11 g	Jellies	60 g	0 g
Mayonnaise (regular)	1 T	8 g	Mustard	1 T	0 g
Peanut butter	1 T	10 g	Blackberry conserve	1 T	0 g
Chocolate biscuit	1 biscuit	5.5 g	Plain biscuit	1 biscuit	3 g
Full cream milk	250 mL	10 g	Lite milk	250 mL	3.5 g
Yogurt	200 g	8 g	Low-fat yogurt	200 g	2 g

tub, you will need to double the calorie quantities listed per serving in the nutrition information. As a start, the 100-g (3.5-oz) serving size is a useful way to compare labels. It can be helpful to check whether products are endorsed by reputable organizations, such as the American National Heart Foundation.

Labels can be literally quite hard to read, especially on smaller products. When you go shopping, have reading glasses or a magnifying glass with you. The language used on labels also can be confusing. When looking for the fat content in a product, there are many pitfalls. Remember that ingredients may be listed as a variety of different types—for example, oil, palm oil, virgin or extra virgin oil, butter, cocoa butter, Copha, lard, dripping, cream, whole milk solids, cheese, cooking margarine, animal shortening, mono-, di-, or triglycerides. Also, "fat free" doesn't mean "no fat"; it only means that a product contains no more than 1.5% fat. "Low fat" means that the food must contain no more than 3% fat. This is sometimes written as "97% fat free"—remember that this relates to a single portion or serving, not to the whole package. Similarly, "cholesterol-free" or "low cholesterol" does not mean "fat free." Cholesterol is mainly found in foods that contain animal products; other fats come from vegetable products, such as olive, coconut, peanut, or safflower oil. "Toasted," "baked," or "creamed" usually means that fat has been added in the preparation of the product. "Lite" or "light" does not always refer to reduced fat; it may mean reduced salt or calories or lighter texture or color.

Assessing sugar content also has its pitfalls. "No added sugar" or "unsweetened" tells us that extra sugar hasn't been added. Some of these foods or drinks, such as fruit juices, already have a naturally high sugar content. Sugar can also masquerade under other names like dextrose, fructose, glucose, invert sugar, and maltose. Sometimes these ingredients are listed separately to make us think that there is less sugar; for example, 15 g of sugar might be listed as 5 g of fructose, 5 g of invert sugar, and 5 g of glucose.

Food Preparation

Food preparation for meals is another time when it is important to make disruptive choices. When other people at home are supportive, they can be enlisted to help in the preparation phase. Plan the menu together, and, if possible, prepare it together so that household members get to understand that healthy eating is really all right. Also, we can encourage our family to buy us healthy cookbooks and disrupting utensils, such as steamers, as presents.

Rotate healthy cooking methods, for example steaming some days, then microwaving, broiling, and dry baking other days. When I am "forced" to fry food in oil or deep fry, I use spray-on oil and cut the food into larger pieces so less oil is absorbed. I get bored with the same low-fat substitutes, so I rotate low-fat substitutes in recipes; for instance, I use low-fat, unsweetened soya milk rather than always low-fat cows' milk. Rather than thickened flour or butter-based sauces, I use a variety of herbs, spices, and seasonings that replace energy-rich sauces; for example, I use chili and fennel in dishes— both increase taste and increase food elimination at the same time.

Messages to Keep

Whether just starting out to achieve a healthy weight for the first time or trying again after several attempts, the path to achieving healthy weight can seem never ending—and it is. Vigilance about healthy eating is as important as sleep.

> *We live in a changing world. We should expect no less from our weight management.*

To achieve a healthy weight and stay there, it is important to remember that:

- Healthy eating should be part of a multifaceted disruptive program, for example, combine healthy eating with activity and lifestyle changes. And we need to change the sequences and components as soon as we start to feel they might not be working for us or we become bored.

- We can look forward to long-term success that is easy to maintain. Dietary disruptions should be made at a manageable pace. A disruptive program that is gradual and realistic is what we always have to have in our minds. Healthy eating strategies will become second nature, sustainable, and capable of being incorporated into everyday life—once the old unhealthy ones are permanently disrupted.

- Understanding how weight is lost is important: up to 5 kg (over 10 lb) in three months, 10 kg (over 20 lb) in 12 months, and down to our best BMI sustained for 10 years. Now that's a goal!

My Top 10 Tips for Disruptive Dieting

1. Vary the diet you are on in some way regularly for years. I varied mine every month (different foods, combinations, or overall diet) every month for 10 years. Over the years, I found the range of healthy foods and drink I could live with for years, not just months.

2. Sight and smell are important senses connected to eating. Always make sure you like the look and smell of what you are about to eat. It reinforces your choices.

3. Have a weight-loss diary (or album or scrapbook), in which you store diets and foods that work for you. It can be daunting to keep those notes at first out of fear you will fail and have to look at the failures, but it will be worth it and help your journey to success.

4. Choose a diet where you can keep count easily, whether that means fat, calories, or other factors. You can also look for free apps that will keep count for you. One popular free program is MyFitnessPal.com, and it calculates calories, fat, protein, carbohydrates, and other factors you can choose, also keeping a tally for the entire day.

5. Visualize stopping eating before you start. What will I leave on my plate? How full should you aim for? It is a bit like a disruptive weight prayer.

6. If you have to eat out, have something that makes you feel less hungry before you leave home, such as carbonated water.

7. Move your dish out of reach when you decide you've eaten enough. If that is not possible, put your napkin over the plate so that you don't have to look at the food. That also stops other people commenting on what you have/have not eaten. Sometimes when I really feel my resolve is weakening, I spill some drink onto my plate—that really makes it look unappetizing.

8. Convince yourself that "something doesn't agree with me." For instance, you don't like cake.

9. Limit any "fails" to small portions no more than once a week. Two or three bites and ditch it. You may ultimately realize that those couple or few bites satisfy the need; any later ones don't taste any better or make you any happier.

10. Don't stop rotating your type of diet and length of the time you stay on it. Disruptive dieting should be exciting and fun. When you "get" how to do it, try and teach it to others!

Notes

1. http://www.nhs.uk/chq/pages/1126.aspx?categoryid=51
2. https://ndb.nal.usda.gov/ndb/search/list?qlookup=&qt=&manu=&SYNCH RONIZER_URI=%2Fndb%2Fsearch%2Flist&SYNCHRONIZER_TOKEN =72506d10-adf4-43ca-acbc-3f5c78047efc&ds=
3. https://cenegenics-boca.com/wp-content/uploads/2016/04/Consultant.pdf
4. http://www.nature.com/ijo/journal/vaop/ncurrent/full/ijo2016156a.html
5. http://ajph.aphapublications.org/doi/full/10.2105/AJPH.2016.303326
6. http://journals.plos.org/plosone/article?id=10.1371/journal.pone.0161297
7. https://health.gov/dietaryguidelines/2010
8. http://guidelines.diabetes.ca/browse/chapter11
9. http://www.sciencedirect.com/science/article/pii/S000282230902094X
10. http://www.nejm.org/doi/full/10.1056/NEJM199801083380212#t=article
11. https://www.scientificamerican.com/article/science-reveals-why-calorie -counts-are-all-wrong
12. http://www.mdpi.com/2072-6643/8/1/45/htm
13. http://www.sciencedirect.com/science/article/pii/S0261561416000443
14. http://ajcn.nutrition.org/content/103/2/305.short
15. http://advances.nutrition.org/content/7/5/866.short
16. http://pediatrics.aappublications.org/content/128/1/201.full
17. http://www.nature.com/ijo/journal/v39/n11/full/ijo201596a.html
18. http://www.sciencedirect.com/science/article/pii/S0195666314004206
19. http://www.andjrnl.org/article/S2212-2672(13)01128-3/abstract

20. http://www.racgp.org.au/afp/2016/januaryfebruary/cutting-through-the-paleo-hype-the-evidence-for-the-palaeolithic-diet

21. http://gph.sagepub.com/content/3/2333794X16669014.full

22. https://www.niddk.nih.gov/health-information/health-topics/weight-control/choosing-safe-successful-weight-loss-program/Pages/choosing-safe-successful-weight-loss-program.aspx

23. http://www.fasebj.org/content/30/1_Supplement/405.1.short

24. https://www.researchgate.net/publication/311095660_Impact_of_the_Swap_It_Don't_Stop_It_Australian_National_Mass_Media_Campaign_on_Promoting_Small_Changes_to_Lifestyle_Behaviors

25. https://www.science.gov/topicpages/e/effective+weight+loss

26. http://www.sciencedirect.com/science/article/pii/S0091743516301530

27. http://bmcpublichealth.biomedcentral.com/articles/10.1186/s12889-016-3112-z

28. http://www.thelancet.com/pdfs/journals/lancet/PIIS0140-6736(16)31338-1.pdf

29. http://www.nature.com/ijo/journal/vaop/naam/abs/ijo2016175a.html

30. http://circ.ahajournals.org/content/125/9/1157.full

31. http://onlinelibrary.wiley.com/doi/10.1111/obr.12366/full

32. http://www.mdpi.com/2072-6643/8/6/354/htm

33. http://journals.lww.com/jbisrir/Abstract/2015/13100/Intermittent_fasting_interventions_for_the.8.aspx

34. http://nutritionreviews.oxfordjournals.org/content/71/2/67.abstract

35. http://ajph.aphapublications.org/doi/full/10.2105/AJPH.2016.303326

36. http://www.thelancet.com/journals/lancet/article/PIIS0140-6736(16)31338-1/fulltext?rss%3Dyes=

37. http://circ.ahajournals.org/content/133/2/187.short#page

38. http://link.springer.com/article/10.1007/s13679-015-0184-5

39. http://psycnet.apa.org/psycarticles/2012-32646-001

40. http://onlinelibrary.wiley.com/doi/10.1111/j.1467-789X.2010.00769.x/full

CHAPTER THREE

The Ins and Outs of Our Bodies

Our digestive system is just like any transit system: It is a route to get products to where they have to go. There are two parts to it. What we put into it—our diets (and these have been discussed in Chapter 2) and what happens along the way—which is the focus of this chapter. We will travel through the absorption and excretion processes in our intestines, and, using scientific evidence, I will show you the ways of making our excretions healthier and weight disruptive. We will also have a look at our intestinal "residents," like bacteria, and "visitors," including laxatives, and how they can retrain and maintain healthy throughput along our food highways, when used responsibly.

My View

What we put out of our bodies is as essential to healthy weight maintenance as what we put into them. It's about healthy bowels, bladders, and skin. I know what I need to do to make sure my output is as healthy as my input. I got overweight by being very efficient in extracting everything out of what I ate. I am just as efficient in excreting what I don't need in my Western world diet where food is in excess of my needs. For example, there is no right number, shape, size, or frequency of bowel movements, but I know what is right for me, and that varies depending on what I am doing and what I eat and drink. Unlike eating, the more I move my bowels in a healthy way, the better. Regular use of products that increase intestinal throughput, such as natural laxatives like herbal teas, can help retrain our intestines for healthy excretion.

In previous chapters, we have looked at ways to limit and select what we put into our mouths; that is only the first part of our food handling. The processing of food and liquids occurs through all the parts of our digestive tract. First, we need to prepare food and drink for transportation to the areas where it is best absorbed—the stomach and the small and large intestines; then we need to break it down and absorb what we need and finally get rid of what we don't need. Our mouths are responsible for reducing what we have eaten to a small enough size to go down our esophagus—the food tube that travels through the chest to the stomach. In that tube, enzymes and bacteria begin to break down food.

> *A disruptive "eating wardrobe" should have utensils that allow only small portions to get into our mouths, like small forks and spoons, chopsticks . . . and outdoor gloves.*

An important step in disruptive eating is to challenge our eating and drinking habits. There have been lots of theories about how to use our mouths to disrupt our ingestion of food that is in excess to our needs. Table 3.1 separates the realities from the beliefs.

In Chapter 2, we learned a lot about what we eat. In this chapter, I want to first focus on how, where, when we eat, as well as the best means to turn our usual fatty ways into methods more helpful to our bodies and minds in the long term.

Geena

Geena weighed 267 lb and was 5'6" tall. She had plateaued at this weight, going up and down a couple of pounds for about a year, after having gained significant weight over the previous decade, despite multiple diets. In the past year alone, she had dieted five times. Geena often skipped meals, restricted calories and fats, and attempted any fad diets that caught her interest. Despite all these attempts, she overate at least once a day. Geena lived with her husband of 10 years and her teenage daughter. Geena was ashamed of her eating patterns. She would always try to find some excuse not to eat with the family because she was ashamed.

Together, we developed habits to help her disrupt her toxic eating patterns. First, she had to realize that what we were going to do was no more disruptive than what she already was putting herself through. Just as she got dressed to start each day and carefully selected what she wore to hide her weight, she needed to carefully get ready to eat. What she was going to put in her mouth was as important as what she chose to wear. In the beginning, an important habit was to get her an eating "wardrobe" that could help her disrupt the way she put food into her mouth. Wherever possible, she had to choose utensils that limited the amount of food she could take in one mouthful. She bought an assortment of chopsticks, small

Table 3.1   Beliefs and Realities about Dieting

Belief	Reality
Eating slowly will help us lose weight.	*Wrong:* It makes no difference.[a]
Eating slowly can help us maintain our weight loss.	*True:* It is useful in weight control, not loss. It won't help us lose weight, but it can be part of a process to keep us stable once each disruption phase is complete.[b]
Eating quickly will put on weight.	*Partially True:* Yes, but only in children and infants. Children who eat quickly are likely to put on up 2.8 kg (6.17 lb) more weight than children who eat slowly. Once we reach middle age, it makes no difference.[c]
Eating with a fork rather than a spoon will help us lose weight.	*Partially True:* Eating with a fork will not help us lose weight. But overweight people are more likely to eat with a spoon to shovel food into their mouths. It seems that foods are more appealing if eaten with a spoon.[d]
Drinking more water helps us lose weight.	*True:* Drinking water can often be a substitute for snacking.[e]
Not drinking with a meals helps us lose weight.	*Partially True:* Drinking too many high-energy drinks at any time puts on weight, so drinking them when we eat will, of course, put on weight. Drinking low-energy drinks, such as water or mineral water, with meals has no effect on weight.
Restraining our eating helps us lose weight.	*True:* it probably the best overall strategy to lose weight during eating.

[a]http://onlinelibrary.wiley.com/store/10.1002/oby.20842/asset/oby20842.pdf;jsessionid=F46F26E10361DFAC1149CA59EAC00DE4.f02t03?v=1&t=j9a6c7yc&s=48028d93bad4944e179e71a1f1a728638ad0da54

[b]http://www.nature.com/ijo/journal/v39/n11/full/ijo201596a.html

[c]https://www.cambridge.org/core/journals/public-health-nutrition/article/speed-of-eating-and-3-year-bmi-change-a-nationwide-prospective-study-of-mid-age-

[d]http://www.sciencedirect.com/science/article/pii/S095032931530015X

[e]http://ajcn.nutrition.org/content/early/2013/06/26/ajcn.112.055061.short

spoons, small forks, and outdoor gloves. The latter prevented her hands from being substitutes for eating utensils; anything she could eat directly with her hands was off-limits. When she felt that she was weakening and about to grab something from the fridge, she put on a pair of dirty outdoor gloves! When eating at home, she would set aside something small for that snack later on to reward myself.

Because of her job, she had to eat out a lot, and this made her very anxious. We developed a number of eating-out habits that she could draw on. If people were watching what she ate, making her anxious, she would always have a napkin to throw on her plate to cover her food. A napkin to cover the plate was also useful for those times when she was full enough but felt she was weakening. Disrupting her plate by forming parts that were no-go zones was another strategy. When the food was placed in front of her, Geena would mentally divide the plate into sections and make a pact not to eat a certain section. In the beginning, it didn't matter what was in that section; it was just to start the practice. Gradually, she moved to placing more and more high-calorie, low-nutrition foods into that zone. She didn't engage in discussions about what everyone was going to eat or look at what they were eating. It would only make for a comparison, and that made her anxious. When picking something from a menu, she practiced disruption, like randomly picking something on the menu from the healthy eating section or ordering the same as someone else who has chosen to eat healthily. Bread on a side plate was always a problem, so she decided to make it unappealing by spilling water on it to make it too soggy to eat. Water was useful in other ways. Geena always asked for sparkling mineral water over tap water because they tend to bring it sooner (so they can sell more?), and she could fill herself up with the carbonated water before eating. If she found herself in an eating frenzy or just thinking too much about food, she took a break to visit the bathroom.

The most important habit was to be kind to herself if she hadn't succeeded in some kind of disruption but be strong enough to say to herself that next time she wouldn't make the same mistake.

Choose mineral water over tap water in restaurants because they tend to bring it sooner and it is filling, so it helps reduce appetite with no associated calories.

The mouth is also a place for excretion. In Chinese medicine, vomiting or purging is an accepted way of expelling fluids that are blocked in the upper body.[1] Purging is fraught with extremely harmful side effects because the stomach is full of strong acids, and they come back up with the food. Vomiting is not the natural direction of food travel in the body, and our esophagus, mouth, and teeth are not prepared for all that acid. We can end up losing the enamel on our teeth, burning or tearing our esophagus, and even getting food into our lungs. So vomiting is not a recommended way of excreting excess foodstuffs. Excess vomiting is just as addictive as eating and is common in people who binge eat, especially among sexual minorities.[2]

After being swallowed, our food spends some time digesting in our stomachs. The size of our stomach, and how much it can increase, determines how fast it works to process food. The larger and faster our stomachs can expand, the more likely they are to act on food. How quickly they can empty the food into the intestines is also important. Surprisingly, stomach size isn't related to body size. Overweight women have the same range of stomach sizes as women at normal range weight. Even women who binge have the same size stomachs as lean women. When food first enters the stomach, the top of it relaxes and expands to hold the food. Then the stomach muscles start pushing the food against the opening to the small intestine (called the pylorus) in order to open it. The pylorus then opens to gradually allow our stomach empty.

As we put on weight, hormones in our stomach designed to minimize the amount of food we absorb stop working effectively.

There is no fixed amount of time the stomach takes to empty. Also, as we'd expect, it varies between solids and liquids. For liquid meals, emptying occurs immediately and with accelerating speed. Solid meals sit in the stomach for about 30 minutes before emptying starts, and it empties at a steadier pace. Stomach hormones control the rate of digestion, appetite, and whether we feel hungry. For example, altering the transit time through our stomach can have a big impact on our appetite and whether we feel full or not. Over time, as we put on weight, our stomachs get used to these hormones, and they don't work as effectively. Some studies have shown that diet can influence the effect of these hormones—but only in the short term or if the diet is maintained. Obese patients put on caloric restriction (a very low-calorie diet) for four days can regain the effect these hormones, and this is maintained for over a year on the diet. However, this effect is lost after one month if the diet isn't maintained.

Several different types of hormones are in our stomach. One group of hormones slows down emptying from our stomach. The most well-known of these hormones is leptin. Leptin, along with cholecystokinin (CCK) and peptide YY (PYY), decreases appetite and slows down stomach emptying to increase the sense of fullness. As our stomach doesn't actually take in much food through its walls, the role of these hormones is to send messages to our brain and body that we have eaten enough.

Other hormones in the stomach stimulate appetite and cause our stomach to empty faster. Faster emptying means less of a feeling of fullness and so a greater likelihood of our continuing to eat.[3] The most well-known of these hormones are ghrelin, glucagon-like peptide (GLP-1), and motilin.

From the stomach, our digesting food moves to the small intestine, where we absorb 95% of all our nutrients. The span it takes food and fluids to travel through our small intestines, called intestinal transit time, is important because it determines the amount of nutrients we absorb. It is a complex process. The muscles in the small intestine that push nutrients through have two types of actions. When we eat, the intestines are in a feeding pattern that is unpredictable, and its speed depends on the amount and type of food ingested. This allows for the food to travel through at a pace that gives enough time for proper digestion and absorption. When we are not eating, there is a fasting pattern that has a regular series of cycles of muscles contracting and relaxing. These muscles are responsible for clearing out the food still there. Obese patients are thought to have altered, slower fasting patterns, which means more absorption occurs during noneating times.

The longer it takes to move the food along the intestines, the more we take in and gain weight. The reverse is also true: Shorter transit times mean less time for absorption, and consequently weight loss is more likely. The type of food we eat also affects the transit time. Persistently high-fat diets increase the length and number of cells in the small intestine and that can increase our absorption of fat.

The bacteria in our intestines that help us absorb nutrients also have a role in moderating our weight. Overweight people have more bacteria in their small intestines, and these bacteria can change the patterns of contractions in the small intestine. In overweight people with other health problems, such as irritable bowel syndrome, these contractions can further slow transit and increase absorption. It is really important to keep the bowel healthy and the contents moving along through it.

James

James is an obese teenager who frequently had diarrhea, especially after eating spaghetti, which was his favorite food. He was quite pale, and blood tests showed he had low levels of iron in his body. He was given some iron tablets and told to eat less spaghetti and more red meat. His diarrhea stopped, but he continued to put on weight (20 lb over six months). James has celiac disease, which means the gluten in most carbohydrate products, such as bread and pasta, is toxic to his small intestine. With all that diarrhea and inability to tolerate pasta, you might think that James would have lost weight, not gained it. The reverse is true. Celiac disease destroys parts of the small intestine, and the remaining sections then work harder, overcompensate, and extract more calories than necessary. That is why James was putting on weight despite changing his diet.[4] Once we started him on a gluten-free diet, he was able to experience weight changes that matched his disruptive practices.

Again, healthy weight is very much a part of maintaining healthy bowel movements. When the remnants of what we eat enter our large intestines, they mainly comprise waste products to be excreted and water to be absorbed. Our large bowel absorbs up to 2 L a day. It lets only 100 ml through with the stools. Our large intestine has three muscles that run along its length and contract involuntarily in reaction to the stimulus of food and fluids. They run lengthways along the bowel and are positioned at 4, 7, and 11 o'clock around the outside of the bowel. Inside the bowel are thousands of frond-like projections that absorb water and salts. The remaining waste products are pushed along by the muscles. The large intestine is only sensitive to expansion and has very little capacity to register pain. That is why we must be consciously aware to make sure it is emptied completely and regularly.

> *If we haven't trained our muscles well when we were young, the walls of our large intestine blow out like balloons and become garbage dumps for our waste products.*

When we are young, our intestinal muscles are strong and can contract efficiently. The muscles respond not only to the quantity of food and liquids passing through but also to the types. High-fat diets can slow down the transit of waste and foods through our large intestines.[5] A slow-moving bowel is unhealthy and can cause problems later in life. When we are young, fiber can help speed up the transit again. Fiber is indigestible and provides the bulk to make the intestinal muscles work harder to push out stools. To prevent the fiber from clogging up in our bowels like cement, we need to take in enough fluid to keep everything moving. As we get older, the muscles and the walls of our bowel get weaker. If we haven't trained our muscles well when we were young, the walls of our large intestine blow out like balloons (diverticula) and become garbage dumps for our waste products. This is called diverticulosis. At this stage, it is too late to use fiber to maintain regular clearing out because the damage is already done.

Kim

I met Kim at a training course I was running at Harvard on leadership for women health professionals. She was a physician who had come from

Korea to attend the course. She told me about her experiences in a trial to modify her gut microbiome. Before the trial, she had a BMI of 23.2 kg/m^2, which is overweight for Asians. She attended a family practice clinic in Seoul and had a consultation with a dietician, who told her that the main dietary causes of her overweight were alcohol and meat. Twice a week, she would go out with her friends and have the equivalent of 10–12 standard glasses of alcohol. She also worked late at the hospital and would often get take-away meals, usually including some kind of fish or meat in a sandwich, followed by an ice cream.

With the help of her dietician, she disrupted the heavy protein intake and increased vegetable intake. She also reduced her alcohol to six standard drinks once a week. Compared to her starting weight, she had lost 3 kg after two months.

To that point, there was nothing unusual in her story. But then she told me how the clinic had tested her feces before and after the diet. *Firmicutes* was the main microorganism before the intervention (70% of total microbiota), whereas after the intervention, *Bacteroidetes* (30%) and *Prevotella* (40%) were most common.

The human body contains trillions of microorganisms that inhabit our bodies after birth and change throughout our lifetime. They are called gut microbiota. We have more than 10 times the number of bacterial cells in our bodies than all of our other cells. A wide range of these organisms live in our bowels. The human gut microbiome, or the microorganisms living in the gut, and their genes contain more than a hundredfold the number of genes that we do. These microorganisms help us sort out what we have taken in; they help break down what we eat into what we need to absorb and what we should treat as waste products. They also help us in making the vitamins that we need. Even though the exact mechanisms linking gut microbiota to obesity are not well understood, we do know that these microbiota can increase energy production from our diet and change fatty tissue to white—both of which contribute to obesity. Changing these organisms to less energy-efficient ones and lessening the time they get to interact with what we eat and drink can be helpful in moderating our weight.

Our gut microorganisms go through a natural life cycle. We start out life in the womb without any microbes. Then, during childbirth, if it is a natural childbirth, we are exposed to our mother's vaginal microbes. Babies born through Caesarian section also get their bacteria from their mother—but usually from their skin. Feeding is another source of microorganisms and breast-fed babies get different ones from formula-fed babies. Our microbes change again when we start eating solid foods. After that, our gut microbes remain relatively unchanged until we get old, when they change again. The four main families of bacteria are *Firmicutes*, *Bacteroidetes*, *Actinobacteria*, and *Proteobacteria*.[6]

Our mouths and our large intestines contain 10 times as many bacteria as our stomachs and small intestines. The microorganisms in the mouth help break down the food, and those in the large intestine are more involved with helping us absorb what we need by breaking down fiber and proteins.[7] We can now exchange our obesity microorganisms for ones that are not so prone to support excess weight. This is good news. Until now, however, such an exchange has been shown to work only in extreme dieting where obesity-generating microorganisms are replaced with other "lean" ones. However, once these diets are stopped, the old microorganisms come back. This is good evidence that disrupting our diets can help us achieve lifelong changes.[8]

There are many ways to introduce lean organisms into our bodies. We can buy probiotics or prebiotics anywhere. Both are chemicals that are supposed to induce the growth of lean microorganisms. Currently there is no evidence that these probiotics or prebiotics actually change the organisms in our intestines. The problem with ingesting these lean microorganisms is that our digestive tracts are designed to break down what we eat—for example, by strong acids in the stomach that may destroy them first—so they may not reach our large intestines. Certainly, they are worth trying as part of a larger disruptive process.

To bypass the problem of breakdown, other approaches have focused on introducing these microorganisms at the other end of our intestinal tract. Studies have begun on fecal transplants. These transplants come from either our own stools, which are mixed with lean microorganisms, or the stools of lean individuals who have the lean microorganisms. Both types are processed and implanted into our intestines from the bottom by a colonoscope or from the top by an endoscope. While fecal transplants from lean individuals can change our stool microorganisms, the long-term effects on weight have not yet been proven. Researchers are now working on freeze-drying these transplants in order to be able to take them as tablets so that they can withstand possible destruction along with way, such as from strong acids in the stomach.[9]

> *Lean individual fecal transplants change stool microorganisms, but the long-term effects on weight have not been proven.*

Laxatives

Excretion is essential to achieve and maintain healthy weight. No matter what we put into our bodies, our bodies have built-in survival mechanisms working to extract the greatest possible nutrition/energy from what travels through. That is why it is important to work as hard on what we remove from our bodies as we do on what we put into them. Though there is little supporting research, the commonly held normal frequency of stools ranges from one stool every three days to three times a day and gets less as we get older and our intestines get tired. For each of us, we are used to our own normal number of times. When we start dieting, we take in less food, so we have less to excrete, and our bowel movements generally become less often. This can make the bowels lazy. Altered bowel movements are frequent in people who are overweight, often beginning in childhood. One in five obese children suffer from constipation, and that is double the number of healthy weight children who suffer from constipation.[10]

We rarely talk about our bowel movements outside of a consultation with our doctor. The term "constipation" can cover a range of problems associated with excretion including very hard stools, straining when going to the toilet, and infrequent bowel movements. Women are more likely than men to complain of constipation and infrequent defecation. African Americans are also more likely to let their doctors know that they have a problem.[11] While constipation is the more common problem for obese people, they are also more likely to suffer from diarrhea than healthy weight people.[12]

In the short term, laxatives can be useful when we are changing our weight-loss activities, such as changing from one diet to another or after bariatric surgery. Often, it takes time for our intestines to adjust to new food compositions, and laxatives in the short term can help maintain healthy bowel habits. Every time we think of changing our diet, we need to consider the effect on our bowels and regulate them for the new disruption.

Laxative "water weight loss" returns as soon as we drink any fluids and the body rehydrates.

In the longer term, laxatives are not a useful way to maintain weight loss. They act in the large intestine to speed up our excretion of water, minerals, electrolytes, and indigestible fiber. This "water weight loss" returns as soon as the body rehydrates.

The common medicinal laxatives are grouped into five categories: stimulants, stool softeners, bulkers, lubricants, and water absorbers. Like any part of the disruptive process, we need to change and disrupt the type of laxatives we use to prevent our bodies getting used to them and having long-term side effects. Table 3.2 shows the range of available laxatives and how they work.

Other Excretions: Sweat, Breath, and Gas

Water makes up about 60% of the human body. Rapid weight loss can always be achieved by decreasing the amount of water in our bodies; however, invariably it comes back. Each liter of water in our body weighs 1 kg, so rapid water loss is a well-known but dangerous technique that is nonetheless used by athletes who compete in sports where weight is important, such as wrestlers, boxers, jockeys.

The body requires at least 1.5 L (six and a half glasses) of water a day to function properly, including keeping the kidneys functioning. By restricting our water intake, we can easily change our body weight by 1.5 kg (3.3 lb) per day. But it won't last, and water restriction has its own health effects.

Water is also required to carry away the by-products of our body. It does this by becoming urine. Depending on how much we drink, we produce 1–2 L (4.5–9 glasses) of urine a day. Each liter of urine weighs 1 kg (2.2 lb). So we can alter our body weight daily just by increasing our urine excretion. That is how so-called water pills work.

Other systems in the body also excrete water. Skin is our largest organ and is responsible for a variable amount of excretion of water. We can sweat out water and salt at a maximum rate of 2,000 mL/hour (nearly 9 glasses). The daily water loss in sweat is quite variable: from 100 to 8,000 mL (half a glass to 32 glasses, or 16 pounds) per day. So our daily weight can change quite radically depending on how much we sweat. Sauna use can cause a loss of up to 2 L a day, or 2 kg (4.14 lb).[13] Such a quick loss can be very rewarding for someone starting to lose weight, but it is not sustainable, and the weight is quickly put back on as our bodies readjust our fluid balance.

The air we breathe is also quite "wet." We need the water in our breath to lubricate our breathing systems. The amount of water we breathe out is roughly 250–350 mL per day which is equivalent to 0.25–0.35 kg (0.55–0.77 lb).

Passing Gas

The bacteria in our intestines that help us digest our food also produce a lot of gas—up to 10 L a day—most of which is taken back into the body. Each liter of gas weighs very little, 0.2 g (less than 1 oz), but it occupies a lot of space in our intestines and can add to our feeling of fullness.

Table 3.2 Types of Laxatives and How They Work

Type of Laxative	How They Work	Examples
Stimulants	Cause the intestines to contract.	Correctol Dulcolax Senokot
Stool softeners	Help mix fluid into stools to soften them.	Colace Docusate Surfak
Bulk-forming agents	Absorb fluid in the intestines, making stool bulkier and, in turn, triggering the bowel to contract and push out the stool.	Citrucel FiberCon Konsyl Metamucil Serutan
Lubricants	Coat the stool, helping it hold in fluid and pass more easily.	Fleet Zymenol
Osmotic agents	Help the stool retain fluid.	Cephulac Phospho-Soda Milk of Magnesia Miralax Sorbitol
Chloride channel activators	Causes the intestines to secrete chloride, leading to increased water secretion and soft stools.	Lubiprostone (Amitiza®)
High-fiber foods	Absorb fluid in the intestines, making stool bulkier, which in turn triggers the bowel to contract and push out stool.	Figs Flaxseed Plums
Fruits, teas, vegetables	Accelerate transit through the small intestine to minimize absorption.	Chilis Pu'er Bekunis Radishes

Note: Laxatives containing phenolphthalein should not be used because they may cause cancer. Most laxatives sold in the United States do not contain phenolphthalein. Nevertheless, always check the ingredients on the medicine's package or bottle. Warning: Longer-term laxative use causes the loss of water, minerals, electrolytes, which can be dangerous.

Source: https://www.niddk.nih.gov/health-information/digestive-diseases/constipation/treatment

Farting is important to maintaining a healthy weight and body. Bloating, which is the result of retaining too much gas, can cause pain and make clothes feel tighter than they should. That sends the wrong messages to our brains about what we are achieving in weight loss.

Though there are no scientific studies, some researchers suggest that between 10 and 20 farts per day is the usual range with a volume of anywhere between two and six glasses worth. Imagine not excreting that and carrying that around in our abdomens after every meal. The retention of gas and bloating are more of a problem for obese people, probably because the microorganisms in the gut of overweight people are less efficient at recycling the gas. They are also problematic for older people because, as our intestinal muscles age and get surrounded by a lot of fatty tissue, the movement of what we eat and drink changes in our bodies. Gases accumulate more, and our abdomens blow up like balloons.

Traditionally, it was culturally permissible for men to fart but not for women. Freud labeled the pain from gas trapped under the rib cage by fashionably tight corsets "hypochondriasis," which translates from the original Greek as "a problem under the rib cage." But the term has evolved into something more psychiatric and socially unacceptable.

Our current society has made farting in public impermissible—mainly because of the accompanying sounds and smells. That is perhaps part of the reason why medical conditions such as excess bloating and irritable bowel disease have developed. Gas expansion in a confined space is painful. With meters of bowel to twist around the air bubbles, it is no wonder that bloating occurs and is difficult to ease. Even when it does shift, the bowel has been stretched and distended. Like any muscle, it is bound to be painful, making the bowel irritable, perhaps even chronically, resulting in irritable bowel disease, which is hard to treat, let alone cure. The condition is more common in overweight women than in overweight men—perhaps because it is the norm for men to tighten their belts under, not over, their bellies.[14]

Notes

1. http://s3.amazonaws.com/academia.edu.documents/45833520/Simonis_-_Illness__texts__and_schools_in_Danxi_medicine.pdf?AWSAccessKeyId=AKIAJ56TQJRTWSMTNPEA&Expires=1484919407&Signature=5z9qHI0vnS2J2Gi4OuLAmaMNQ%2Bc%3D&response-content-disposition=inline%3B%20filename%3DIllness_texts_and_schools_in_Danxi_medic.pdf

2. http://onlinelibrary.wiley.com/doi/10.1002/eat.22576/full

3. http://www.gastrojournal.org/article/S0016-5085(14)01423-1/pdf

4. http://www.mdpi.com/2072-6643/6/1/207/htm

5. https://www.ncbi.nlm.nih.gov/pmc/articles/PMC3890396

6. http://www.wageningenacademic.com/doi/pdf/10.3920/BM2014.0104

7. https://lipidworld.biomedcentral.com/articles/10.1186/s12944-016-0278-4

8. https://www.spandidos-publications.com/10.3892/br.2016.649

9. https://www.ncbi.nlm.nih.gov/pmc/articles/PMC5045147

10. http://link.springer.com/article/10.1007/s00383-014-3651-2

11. http://link.springer.com/article/10.1007/BF01537261

12. https://www.ncbi.nlm.nih.gov/pmc/articles/PMC3890396

13. https://www.researchgate.net/profile/Reid_Reale/publication/304529333
_Acute_Weight_Loss_Strategies_for_Combat_Sports_and_Applications_to
_Olympic_Success/links/57759a2b08ae1b18a7dfe1de.pdf

14. http://www.wageningenacademic.com/doi/pdf/10.3920/BM2014.0104

CHAPTER FOUR

Turning Our Heavy Minds into Light Ones

Most of us have tried to lose weight or help someone else to lose weight at some time or other. I tried for years. I succeeded in the short term and failed in the longer term. I could lose weight, even up to 14 kg (30 lb), but it would always creep back on within a year. These failures dominated my mind. Some of the more common negative stories I told myself were: "No matter what I eat or drink, I will still be hungry." "No matter when I eat, I still won't feel full." "No matter what I do, the fat will always win; it's in my genes." Realizing that these thoughts were only the result of a mind trying to assist me the only way it knew how was the first step to reorienting my thoughts.

I reviewed how my patterns began and were seemingly set in stone. Those meals with my grandmother and my parents, feeling so guilty I ate everything on my plate even if I felt full. I became too fat to take part in school sports without ridicule. Though I was very smart, I hated how I looked.

It took many years and many attempts to find a series of paths away from that disastrous obesity highway. Finally, a community of family, friends, and professionals helped me reframe "I have to eat" into "I eat for enjoyment . . . and for life."

Behavioral interventions in obesity come from the belief that, if we can reduce our psychological barriers, then our behaviors will change. The strategies are adapted from those designed to treat people with mental health problems. They are based on the theory that we overeat in response to emotions and that we can't distinguish between emotional reasons for eating and actual, physical hunger. Behavior therapy (BT) provides a set of principles and techniques for helping us modify the eating, activity, and thinking habits that contribute to our excess weight. The strategies are based on looking at the reasons why we put on weight and why we keep it on and on challenging the difficult thoughts that keep us from losing weight. The strategies come in a variety of shapes and sizes, among them metacognitive therapy, acceptance and commitment therapy, mindfulness-based cognitive therapy, dialectical behavior therapy, relaxation therapy, psychodynamic therapy, hypnotherapy, eye movement desensitization and reprocessing, emotion freedom techniques, interpersonal psychotherapy, and compassion-focused therapy targeting. Behavioral therapies can be accessed in a variety of ways: in hospitals or in the community; face to face, by telephone, or online; and with a psychologist, other health professionals, or qualified therapists. In this chapter, we are moving from the why and what of obesity to the who: Let's move from the eating to the eater.

Behavioral therapies disrupt the pathway in our minds from an unhealthy view of weight loss and weight management to a healthy one. The first stage is when we accept that we have to lose weight—no matter how many times we have tried before and failed or only partially succeeded. The second stage is thinking about what changes we can make. We need to review what we have done in the past and what worked and what didn't, as well as which ones we can repeat and which ones we can't. The third step is getting the knowledge and skills to alter our behavior and learning about newer strategies. The next stage is to make changes. Incorporating a series of changes in our daily routine is the final step to the path toward long-term success.

How these treatments work is not always easy to understand, and there are few consistent findings across all the treatments. As we have discovered about most treatments for obesity, standard behavioral weight-control programs are successful in helping us lose weight in the short term; however, nearly all the weight we lose we regain within two to five years. The more intense and frequent interventions in a program, the more likely we will have a greater weight loss and maintain it through to the medium term.[1]

The key components of programs that work include interventions that are at least six months long; trained educators to deliver the educational interventions; wherever possible, one-on-one counselling; and programs that include changes in diets and exercise.[2] On these programs, we can lose approximately 8–10 kg (17–25 lb) or about 8–10% of our initial weight. In programs that last up to a year, approximately 80% of people who begin the program complete it. Weight loss is about 0.4–0.5 kg per week, reaching its peak at about six months.

Behavioral therapies, like diets, work only if we stick to them. The differences with diets are that they often show results quite quickly, that it is acceptable for us to change them when they stop working, and that we are not seen as failures if we do so. Behavioral therapies take longer than diets to show significant weight disruption. Like any disruptive approach, it is important to stay with a strategy until it stops working or until you lose motivation, then move on to another one. No one behavioral therapy has proven to reliably work in the long term—that is why we have to practice disruption with them.

Most behavioral therapies get us to work through a series of steps. First, we have to recognize our patterns. Early on, a food diary record helps us transfer what we know is happening from our minds to something more concrete that we can see. We learn to recognize eating patterns that we need to disrupt. Recording what we eat and drink can help us focus on

Our social networks can act as distracters or facilitators.

specific issues that are causing us difficulty, for example, assessing our hunger level, how our mood might affect our eating or physical activity patterns, or whether the place where we eat is a problem. "Diaries" can take many shapes or forms—they don't have to be written down, and many apps are now available to make monitoring quite simple; for example, a pedometer, which tracks the number of steps we do in a day, is a form of a diary. This self-monitoring can take many forms, but usually it includes maintaining food diaries and activity logs. In a food diary, we write down everything that we eat, add up the number of calories consumed, and/or fat content, where the eating was done, and what was happening/how we were feeling at the time. If we can do this for six months, the research suggests that we will lose weight.

This is one of the key elements in a BT package. It is quite simple, really. If we ignore the signals, we are never going to change. So we have to police ourselves with regular feedback about whether our behaviors are improving, deteriorating, or being maintained. Any diary should let us assess where we are on our disruptive pathway and have the basic format shown in Table 4.1. This is one of the key elements of behavior modification.

Behavioral modification is more sustainable in the long term if we have the support of those around us. When our family members or close others are enlisted to provide ongoing support, we can lose an additional 3 kg (5 lb). Therefore, recording how the people in our social networks are acting is also important; for example, are the people around us helping us or distracting us?

Table 4.1 Example of a Disruptive Diary

Event:	Where:	With whom:	Feelings:	Quantity:	Stage in disruptive cycle:	Ready to plan next strategy:
E.g., eating, exercising, meditating	E.g., home, work, holiday	E.g., alone, helpers, distracters	E.g., optimistic, pessimistic, neutral	E.g., food, drink, physical activity	E.g., beginning, in middle, bored, plateauing	E.g., change diet, behavioral therapy
Lunch	Work	Distracters	Neutral	On low-fat diet	In middle of second cycle (1 month)	No
Power walking after work	With dog	Helper	Optimistic	Power walking every night, yoga once weekly	Plateauing	Yes, exploring gym membership

Diaries just get us to record what we do. It is in our actions that we can experience the changes we make and disconnect the negative wiring that has taken us to an unhealthy place in our minds and bodies. Then, gradually, we can make changes across all the events in our lives. We can realize our potential to behave in a weight-conscious way, such as shopping for the right foods, taking the wrong food purchases out of our shopping baskets, developing a taste for healthier options such as fruits and vegetables. At home, we can exercise our healthy mind too by altering the amount of food served on the table, reducing the size of plates and containers, and concentrating on eating without being distracted by television or reading material.

Mary

In the summer, Mary bought ice cream in large tubs. She always placed it on a prominent shelf in the freezer so that she wouldn't have to bend over to reach it and injure her back. Every time she went to the freezer, she couldn't help seeing it. At first, she told herself she really didn't want any. It was only for the children and her husband. Then she started asking her husband Hal to serve dessert so that she wouldn't have to deal with the ice cream—which was her main snack food weakness. But then when she was tidying up the kitchen, she would take out a few scoops of ice cream straight from the freezer to "reward" herself for maintaining her diet all day. She reassured herself that it was only a few extra calories and that it wouldn't make much difference. She certainly wouldn't tell her husband and even went to great lengths to make the remaining ice cream in the tub look as though it was untouched. Usually that involved eating more ice cream to "level out" the container. Finally, Hal noticed what she was doing, and they discussed ways of dealing with the problem so that Mary wouldn't be either tempted or ashamed. They agreed that, while it was more expensive, they had to replace the tubs with single-serve ice creams. Mary felt that she would be less tempted and also that it would allow her to see the other, healthier things in the freezer.

Mary and her family practiced an acceptance-based strategy. It helped the family to recognize and accept the negative emotions and actions associated with Mary's pains regarding overeating and dieting. Her attitude toward ice cream was just one example. It was important that Mary's family accepted that her painful feelings and thoughts were normal for her. Then the whole family could step back and help Mary detach from the shamed thinking, guilty feelings, and overeating that had brought her both comfort and pain.[3]

The next thing in her diary that Mary wanted to tackle was eating too quickly. She always ate too quickly and never got signals from her stomach to tell her she was full and to stop her overeating. She blamed rushing around after the kids and eating their leftovers, but deep down she knew it was more about how bad she felt about herself and how ashamed and guilty she felt every time she ate. Getting the food down really quickly made the whole process of eating more bearable. We discussed how slowing down her eating could let the hormones of fullness have their say. Using smaller cutlery and forks instead of spoons, cutting up her food as she ate, not in the beginning, and even using the knife and fork the "English" way were all things she agreed to try. Rather than asking the children to take the finished plates away, she took them herself to the kitchen and left them there for the family to wash. She found that doing so not only got her away from the food but also stopped her from grazing at the leftovers and grabbing an ice cream from the freezer.

Mary was following a well-known strategy for weight loss called "goal setting." First, she had to understand that goals were not laws and that she would not be tried by herself or others and a punishment handed out. Goals were her gift to herself, plans she could make and work toward. My job was to help her make sure that they were specific and realistic goals and that she was prepared to change them when they stopped working. Goals need to be specific enough to know exactly what we need to achieve. Instead of setting a general aim like "I want to look better," a goal needs to be more detailed, explaining exactly how this goal will be achieved. So "I want to look better" can be reworked into something we can work with: "I want to look better and have a healthy life, and I will achieve this by losing weight by disruptive strategies until I achieve my desired weight." Two of Mary's specific goals were to stop her ice cream snacking and reduce meal portion size.

There is no point in setting goals if they are unachievable—even if they seem realistic at the time. Many of our weight-loss attempts are cut short because we have unrealistic expectations of what can be achieved in what time frame, and when we fail, we lose our motivation. Often we measure the success or failure of our weight loss by set amounts, such as pounds or kilograms per week. When thinking about how much loss is achievable, we need to remember that in the beginning a realistic rate of weight loss is 0.25–1.0 kg (0.5–2.0 lb) per week, but that slows down over time and is an indication to change our techniques. So "I will achieve this by losing 10% of my body weight in the first year and maintaining my healthy weight for five years" becomes "I will achieve this by losing 10% of my body weight in the first year by losing an average of 2 lb per month for the first six months, then getting to my long-term goal weight within the next two years."

When we plateau, looking at a change in weight as a measure of how we are doing is unhelpful. Because the amount of weight loss is so individual, it is better that we don't compare actual figures with each other; rather, keep in mind that in the beginning of any program, if we behave, we can expect to lose 10% of our initial body weight. When that is achieved, it is time to reflect and to decide whether or when a new strategy is required. Mary decided to tackle the ice cream problem once she plateaued on the current weight-loss program. Goals don't have to be about weight, but weight is the easiest thing to measure. Whatever they are, measurable times and amounts need to be included. Mary set herself time frames for achieving all the steps of her goals: She would completely stop the ice cream snacking problem within three months of agreeing to do so, and she would make sure the disruption of ice cream was still in place at one year.

Not all goals are reached quickly. I usually set short-term goals for periods of up to a month. An example of a short-term goal is to complete a food diary by writing down everything we eat and drink over three days. In this way, we can see where we are going wrong and what foods and beverages need to be targeted. Medium-term goals are the next stepping-stone to achieving long-term goals, and I advise weight dis-

> *At regular intervals, reassess these milestones and disrupt weight-loss activities, if necessary, to keep the process going.*

rupters to expect to achieve them within six months to two years. An example of a medium-term goal is to build up to 30 minutes walking per day over a six-month period. In weight management, the ultimate goal must be long term. Many people say this is achieved when our weight loss is sustained for two years and beyond. An example of a long-term goal is to aim to fit into a clothing that is two sizes smaller than our present size by the time our next birthday comes around and to maintain that loss.

Cognitive behavioral therapy (CBT) has helped me focus on trying to prevent the factors that can cause my weight to increase again after losing it successfully. It is a therapy designed not for weight loss but rather for helping those of us develop a new way of thinking about ourselves. CBT aims to minimize weight regain and helps us develop lifelong strategies and a commitment to effective weight management. This type of therapy doesn't focus on what we lose or have lost; it is more about keeping a stable weight.[4] Through CBT, I have learned to be aware of my risky behaviors—such as stress and boredom—that make me eat when I am not really hungry; to keep myself focused on how much I want to keep these changes going; to develop sound reprogramming approaches so that, when I catch myself in the act of an unhealthy eating behavior, I start thinking about a new alternative, like delaying the trip to the kitchen by 15 minutes and then seeing if I still want to eat; to substitute and add, such as substituting a new (positive) behavior for a less effective one, changing diets when I plateau, or adding a laxative if I blow out one time. All of these steps require regular reflection to review what worked or didn't work so that I can fine-tune the process.

Some techniques sound good but have yet to show any promise. They include cognitive restructuring and adopting positive outlooks therapy, problem-solving therapy, and assertiveness training and stress reduction.[5] It is important to always ask our therapists what can go wrong? After all, therapy is a treatment like any other.[6]

Bob

Bob is in his late fifties and has diabetes and heart problems. He wants to lose weight, but he always puts barriers in place to prevent making changes, such as saying, "Nothing works . . . can't you just give me pills for the rest of my life for my diabetes?" He blames his problem on having to eat out a lot for work. He had tried pausing between courses, drinking sparkling water, and not eating bread while waiting for the meal, but nothing seemed to work.[7] Every consultation, I make suggestions to help him lose weight, and each time he comes to see me, he has gained a bit more weight.

Bob is suffering from "behavioral fatigue," a term used to describe when we are tired of trying and want to give up. When everything seems too hard, we are consciously incompetent to lose weight. The feeling is not uncommon. We all have experienced it. We get a lot of rewards from early weight loss, such as compliments, feeling better, changes on the scales and clothing size, which keep us going. After a while, they stop coming, and our resolve weakens.

The solution is not to stay in the "fatigued" state too long and to view disruption as a life choice. Mindfulness training can help here. Mindfulness is a technique that helps us to "stay in the moment" and not overanalyze what is happening. It involves practicing various forms of meditations and exercises, assisting us to focus on our moment-by-moment experiences, thoughts, and emotions in an open, nonjudgmental way. We all are mindful from time to time. However, by strengthening this process, we can become more aware in a nonjudgmental way of the triggers that make us overeat or eat the wrong foods. Mindfulness training helps us develop skills to accept our lapses as transient, instead of acting on impulses to immediately suppress them by eating. Mindfulness has shown a short-term effect equivalent to most other weight-loss techniques, an average 9 lb lost with the loss sustained for six months.[8] While mindfulness training has not shown any long-term results on weight loss, it has also shown promise in controlling binge eating and in helping us increase our exercise.[9]

Bob needs to let go of the idea that only one strategy will be necessary. He needs to embrace the idea that he is a short visitor to any strategy and that he will always have a range of new strategies to try. It's like buying a pair of shoes. You might be a size 8, but not all size 8 shoes fit or feel comfortable, nor do ones that fit stay comfortable forever. Here are some strategies I used with Bob in no particular order, and we changed them whenever they stopped working.

Think about someone close to you who has recently been diagnosed with a condition other than your own (diabetes) that is related to their being overweight, such as high blood pressure, arthritis, or depression. Keep a mental picture of that person "available" at any time you need it. This technique is called "available thinking." It is a way to keep a reminder with us just like keeping pictures of our families and friends in our minds and our albums.

Bob could act as his own clairvoyant by "foreseeing" what was going to happen if he didn't continue on a disruptive weight management path. He had been there several times before. We arranged a short walk around not only the diabetic clinics but also the vascular clinics for Bob to see what could happen to him if he didn't stick with his weight-loss plans. Talking to some of the people there who were still obese and had major problems from their diabetes, including very poor circulation, decreased eyesight, or being wheelchair bound, gave him good insight.

Stop engaging in magical thinking. We cannot change the circumstances around us by casting a spell and waiting for Harry Potter to wave his wand or bring a magic potion. But we can wave your own inner wands to control ourselves. If a goal has not been reached by the time frame we set for it, we don't need magic to disrupt, reassess, and revise it.

Plan for a marathon, but don't enroll just yet. Early success in all weight management programs tends to make us overconfident that the weight loss will continue to be rapid and permanent. We need to recognize and reward small successes along the way. Short-term goals and a variety of disruptions can help. In the long term, our goal will be reached.

The future always offers hope. Obesity research is evolving. Sometimes there isn't a clear answer. During the last decade, obesity research output has produced at least 55 articles a day—that's over 20,000 a year.

Watch out for the ostrich. It's inside all of us. When things are too negative and the problems seem too large, we tend to bury our heads in the sand like an ostrich. We can lift our heads out of the ground by rotating through a range of strategies, like breaking our goals into healthy small chunks or looking at alternative options. Turn negative concepts into positive ones. Try not to fall into a period of relapse due to a momentary lapse of focus. We need to develop contingency plans or our best intentions could get railroaded. Take a healthy lunch to the game instead of buying a burger or hot dog there. Be prepared for relapses and weight-loss plateaus; these are natural stages on a disruptive weight program. The use of activity and food diaries can help keep us focused.

Sometimes we need to be pushed gently in the right direction and accept that it is the path we should travel. When we do that, it is harder to opt out. If your personality is amenable to group activities, it is always the right time to join a support network, for example a local walking group, as well as regular visits to health professionals.[10] The important thing to remember is that, just like any weight strategy, it needs to be disrupted when it stops working.

A variety of public and private weight-loss therapies are described throughout the book. Most of them offer some kind of behavioral therapy as well as a diet. As a minimum, any process that we chose should provide ready access to information in a variety of ways (e.g. face to face, Internet, telephone, newsletter, book, fact sheets), as well as contact with others who are also in the programs for support in order to share ideas and strategies in overcoming challenges.

Joe

Joe was a patient of mine who had struggled with his weight for many years. He had tried nearly everything. First, he drank diet shakes with no success. Then he went on a diet of protein and green, leafy vegetables. By week 4, he lost 4 kg (9 lb) and stopped dieting. All the weight came back. The following year he tried jogging. By week 8, he lost 2.3 kg (5 lb), but his knees started hurting, and once again put all the weight back on.

Joe would visit me after his attempts failed. Many times, I suggested that Joe join a group. He always refused with some excuse—didn't want to be in a group with just African Americans, he only wanted to be in a group with African Americans, he had too many family commitments, and so on.

After agreeing to take my behavioral test (see Chapter 10), Joe recognized that he was most comfortable as a "team member" and finally agreed to a behavioral therapy group in addition to a program of disruptive weight loss that we devised together. At the time, he was 37 years old and weighed 95.2 kg (210 lb) (BMI 30.1). He attended on a weekly basis for six months. Each session lasted 60 minutes. The sessions began with a private measurement of his weight. Then the group convened, and each person provided a brief report on his or her progress. Joe really liked hearing other people's strategies, successes, and how they overcame problems. He also liked that a new weight management skill was taught in each session. Joe really liked the suggestions about looking at his plate differently. He decided that his whole family would be healthier if they ate off smaller plates, didn't fill them to the edges, and left some food on the plate. For practice, the family would go once a week to the mall and have a meal at the buffet.

Two years later, he came back for a follow-up visit, and his weight had remained steady for a year at 82 kg (181 lb). He had achieved conscious competence (see Chapter 3). He shared a couple of his own strategies with me. Staying focused on how he did something rather than what he wanted to achieve, like thinking about the timing of his meals rather than on whether a particular diet was working or making a commitment to increasing the time he took to eat by 10 minutes and not eating while he was shopping or walking, really helped when he was stuck.

We agreed that I would see him for other health problems but made a pact to review his disruptive strategies as and when needed. Six months later, he was ready to start a long-term disruptive rotational program. He is still losing weight five years later. Joe is the kind of person who works well in groups (see Chapter 10 to help you work that out). Sharing goals in a group is helpful for him—especially when he is starting a new disruptive strategy or when he is on the edge of a plateau and his motivation is flagging.

Because weight management is a widespread concern across the nation, it's more than likely that a group exists in your area or on the Internet. Make contact with a group and attend a few meetings to see how they operate and what resources are required. Or you can form your own through social media, such as Meetup, Facebook, YouTube, Twitter, or by means of a local flyer to let others know that it is happening. Make contact with key people—local doctors, gym instructors, and any others who might know people who might like to join. Leave copies in community centers, post offices, doctors' offices, and libraries. Free or cheap meeting space can often be found in a local church or community center. Some physicians interested in weight management may be open to having a group in their offices, especially after hours. A regular meeting time, like the first Wednesday in every month, makes it easy for people to remember the meeting day. Plan your first meeting carefully. It should really be a time for attendees to introduce themselves, say how they expect to benefit from the group and how they think the group should run. It should also include plans for the next meeting and some time to socialize after the meeting. Future meetings should cover the following issues: What is the purpose of the group? Should it provide emotional and/or practical support? Should it also provide information and/or education? How will the meetings run? How will confidentiality be maintained? How will mutual respect and a nonjudgmental atmosphere be encouraged? What is the membership? Should friends and family members be able to join, or will membership be limited to only those people with weight problems? Will it cost money? What will happen in the meetings? Will the meetings be structured, for example with talks by invited guest speakers, or will they be more of a discussion forum?

Groups periodically experience highs and lows in energy and attendance. It is to be expected. Always be ready to think of ways of keeping the group alive. Checking with members from time to time to review whether the group is meeting their needs can minimize the impact of the lows. Sometimes groups just run their course and need to disband. When that occurs, find new strategies to keep motivated.

Weight-Loss Programs[11]

Inasmuch as long-term success is built on success in a series of short- and medium-term goals, quite often programs focus on short-term gains with the hope that they will translate into longer goals. The long-term efficacy of several types of programs have been reviewed by a group of researchers. The results are shown in Table 4.2.

Many of these therapies can now be delivered over the Internet and smartphones. Virtual contact is more effective than minimal treatment but less effective than face-to-face treatment. For example, twice-monthly counseling, delivered in 15- to 20-minute individual telephone sessions, is as effective as face-to-face group counseling, but it only works if the same counselor is available every time.[12] A typical program might look like this: First, keep a log of what you eat. Then try to eat every meal in only one location and at set times. Start noticing the speed at which you are eating and try to moderate it; for example, count your bites and put down your utensils after every fourth bite. For each day you stick to the program, give yourself a reward, such as setting aside some money to save up for a piece of jewelry or technology. When you have a lapse, don't dwell on it but

Table 4.2   Results of Various Types of Weight-Loss Programs

Weight-Loss Program	Average Weight Changes Sustained for 12 Months	Average Weight Changes Sustained for 2–3 Years
Community-based program	1.8-kg increase	Not measured
Monthly phone calls and written materials	0.95-kg decrease	Not measured
Videotaped resources	4.0-kg decrease	Not measured
Behavioral Therapy after Bariatric surgery	4.4-kg decrease	Not measured
Women attending without husbands	7.4-kg decrease	None
Women attending without husbands but husbands formally agreeing to support them	4.2-kg decrease	None
Women attending with husbands	7.0-kg decrease	None
Monetary commitment	None	
Monetary commitment, lessons, homework	4.0-kg decrease	
Individual behavioral therapy	4.0-kg decrease	
With daily charting	15.4-kg decrease	14.8 kg decrease
Continued therapist contact (fortnightly)	None	
Minimal monitoring	None	
Intensive program (four months)	12.5-kg decrease	Not measured
Exercise class		
Participant-led sessions		

administer a "punishment"; for example, if you eat snack food, take a dose of castor oil.

Before we join any program, key questions need to be answered by the program coordinators. What are the costs and commitments of the program, and do they have some evidence about their success rates? Are program leaders prepared to discuss our involvement not only as participants but also in the decision making so that the program can be tailored to our specific needs and concerns? Is the program flexible enough to provide us with individual diet, motivational, and physical activity goals and to allow for disruption? Can the staff demonstrate expertise in health education, nutrition and counselling? Is there someone who will be especially allocated to help us along the way with personal advice? Are the messages consistent with what we believe and reinforcing enough to trust them? How does the program fit into a long-term strategy of disruption? Can they work with the changes in strategy that we will require?

Notes

1. http://onlinelibrary.wiley.com/doi/10.1002/14651858.CD012114/full
2. http://onlinelibrary.wiley.com/doi/10.1111/j.1467-789X.2007.00351.x/full
3. http://www.sciencedirect.com/science/article/pii/S2352250X14000311
4. https://academic.oup.com/fampra/article/31/6/643/592646/Effectiveness
-of-behavioural-weight-loss
5. https://www.ncbi.nlm.nih.gov/pmc/articles/PMC3263194
6. http://onlinelibrary.wiley.com/doi/10.1002/14651858.CD012114/full
7. http://journals.bmsu.ac.ir/ijmr/index.php/ijmr/article/view/154/155
8. http://onlinelibrary.wiley.com/doi/10.1111/obr.12461/full
9. https://www.ncbi.nlm.nih.gov/pmc/articles/PMC4046117
10. http://www.jmir.org/2013/5/e81/?utm_source=feedburner&utm_medium
=feed&utm_campaign=Feed%3A+JMedInternetRes+(Journal+of+Medical+Inte
rnet+Research+(atom))
11. Glenny A-M, O'Meara S, Melville A, Sheldon TA, et al. The treatment and prevention of obesity: A systematic review of the literature. *Int J Obes* 1997; 21: 715–737.
12. https://www.ncbi.nlm.nih.gov/pmc/articles/PMC3233993

CHAPTER FIVE

Disruptive Movement

Our bodies need to move to stay healthy, but modern technology has reduced much of the need for human movement. Cars reduce the time we spend walking. Machines, such as washing machines, reduce the amount of physical work we do around the house. Home entertainment, such as watching television and using computers, increases our inactive periods. Decreasing physical activity exacerbates overweight and obesity.

> *Exercise stimulates the immune system and works on our fat cells.*

"Physical activity," "exercise," and "physical fitness" are often used interchangeably. This makes the interpretation of the benefits of these activities difficult—especially in weight management. Physical activity is about our daily life activities, such as what we do at work and at home, as well as the sports we play for recreation. It is a broad term describing bodily movements that involve muscle contractions and increase metabolism. Exercise is a more formal part of physical activity. It is planned, structured, and often repetitive. It has more structure and has a goal of getting us or keeping us fit. Physical fitness is how we measure these activities and is determined by our cardiovascular and muscular strength, as well as our age and genetic inheritance. "Physical activity" is a much better term for those of us who are overweight, as it doesn't make us think of elite athletes and bodybuilders.

Like dieting, physical activity can reduce the amount of fat in our cells—more so in our upper bodies.[1] It also stimulates the immune system. Soon, these changes in the immune system will be measurable.[2] The key for weight-loss clients is gradual improvement in our range of physical activities and disrupting our strategies when they stop working or when we lose motivation and can't regain it. There are four categories of physical activity:

1. *Cardiorespiratory physical activity*—The ability to maintain whole body movement for a sustained period of time
2. *Muscular strength*—The ability to maintain the activity of a particular muscle or group of muscles through a series of single activities
3. *Muscular endurance*—The ability to maintain a series of high-intensity muscle contractions without fatiguing
4. *Flexibility*—The ability to move joints through their full range of movement

Within these categories are three levels of intensity:

1. *Light*, such as walking to work
2. *Moderate*, such as swimming or cycling to work
3. *Vigorous*, such as heavy housework or competitive sports[3]

Bill

Bill is 35-year-old office worker of average weight of 160 lb (70–75 kg). His company recently moved into a building with security barriers between the floors, so Bill can no longer use the stairs to go between departments, and he has to take the elevator. Bill recognized that even the most inactive person can gain health benefits from becoming even slightly more active, such as by taking the stairs at work. His wife had already convinced him to walk and to take public transport rather than drive the car or take a cab to work. When added together, all these seemingly little changes make a big difference in the amount of physical activity we do in a day. Using the elevator meant that Bill lost about 2 minutes less walking per hour over an 8-hour day. Over a year, this reduction would add 1 lb (0.5 kg) or, over 10 years, 10 lb (5 kg) to Bill's body weight.

The key to maintaining a high level of physical activity is to think "active" all the time. In the past, it was thought that physical activity of a vigorous nature three or four times a week was all that was needed for good health. That is no longer true.

The best physical activity to start with is walking. Walking does not require expensive equipment. It can be done at any time, even at work as in Bill's case, and is relatively free of potential injury. The impact of walking on the bones and joints is 3.6 times less than the impact of jogging. Start with short walks, say 5 minutes a day, and build up gradually. It can help mark out a course, which you gradually extend. For exercise to help in maintaining our weight loss, we need to walk at a rate that increases our heart rate to 70% of its maximum. A rate above 3 mph (6 km/hr) should do that.

The energy spent on and the intensity of walking can be increased by adding weights to the head, hands, wrists, ankles, or body. However, hand weights, if only held by the side of our body without movement, do not increase weight loss. A pumping action of the arms at a rate of 12 beats per minute, with weights of about 3 lb (1.3 kg), results in a small increase of calories burned (up to 2 calories per minute, depending on body weight). Ankle and backpack weights have less effect.

> *The amount of energy required to achieve any physical activity increases with body size. It is like trying to accelerate a large car versus a small one—there is more of a body to move.*

Walking can be difficult for some of us, especially in extreme weather. For example, if it is too hot, we can overheat and develop rashes and infections in places where our sweat congregates, from armpits and under breasts to groins. Also, walking when we are carrying a lot of weight can be torture on our knees, especially walking on stairs. If Bill had continued only using the stairs as his main form of exercise, his knees may have deteriorated and become painful. That is why he decided to learn how to swim properly. Once he got over his fear of putting his head under water, the buoyancy effect of the water made him feel a lot lighter and made the task of physical activity pleasurable.

Most of the strategies we use to manage weight involve some kind of denial or substitution that has to be managed. Physical activity offers us something positive. It not only raises endorphins—the body's natural "highs"—but also can lead to an improved body shape, which is a bonus. So it is no wonder that there has been a lot of hype about the benefits of physical activity alone in weight management and weight loss. Unfortunately, none of it has been proven conclusively. Some studies show that physical activity is effective especially when we are not fit. However, the relationship between recommended physical activity and obesity in the long term is still unclear.[4] Research has shown both positive and negative effects.[5]

While the long-term benefits of exercise alone are not clear, as in Bill's case, the positive effect of that feeling of lightness can help us to speed up our fitness program, exercise more comfortably, and reduce the risk of injuring ourselves. Cool water conducts the heat away from the body, so working out in the water is good for people who sweat a lot or have hot flushes. Bill was able to be comfortable enough to put his head under water and swim, but for those of us who can't do that, there are buoyancy vests, kickboards, aqua cycles, and swimming fins. We don't need to know how to swim or put our heads under water to benefit from water activities. There are also aqua aero-bics groups or deepwater running and cycling classes for those of us who prefer group water activities.

> *No single strategy works in the long term. We need to keep on disrupting.*

My Story

As a child, I wasn't encouraged to participate in sports or to do much exercise. My activity was limited to riding my bicycle around the local streets until my friends and I had enough coins (from collecting deposit bottles and cans) to buy some sweets from the local shop. I failed the junior school swimming test four times, and, when I nearly drowned the last time, the teachers took pity on me and never asked me to go in the water again.

I was intelligent—and fat. Only schoolwork was important to my par-ents. I was very relieved in my second year of high school to be selected for the debate team, which meant I didn't have to go to do any school sport anymore. The mentally toxic combination of my saying I had period pain (every week) or getting my mother to write a letter to get me out of sport could stop.

When I sustained a disc injury during my later internship, I was forced to rethink my fear of swimming for therapy's sake. With a caring partner and a cousin who swam like a fish, I learned to trust myself in the water. My back improved, and so did my weight and body shape. But I hit a plateau and took up smoking instead and then stopped it. My weight ballooned.

Long-term problems with weight are usually accompanied by other physical health problems, such as heart disorders, diabetes, and arthritis. In my case, it was a disc problem in my back. These conditions can make physical activity difficult. Raising our heart rate too high may be danger-ous if we have heart problems, arthritis in our large joints may make step climbing difficult, and exercising with unstable diabetes may send our sugar levels plummeting. When more than one condition is present, we can be confused by conflicting recommendations and not be able to work out which one to follow. In my case, it was compounded by pain, soreness, depression, and embarrassment. It was then that I realized I needed help to develop a personalized strategy.[6] Even more important was the frequent disruption necessary to deal with the range of my problems.

After I became an academic and started running weight management programs, I realized that body shape influences what activities we can do; rowers, for example, have to have both long arms and legs. My shape was just not suitable for the kind of disruptive physical activity that would help me maintain a healthy weight. My large breasts had a mind of their own when I tried to jog. It was hopeless, and I often gave up after a 5-minute jog. To make matters worse, the battle between glutes and breasts made my back worse.

I went back to what I knew. I got a recumbent cycle (better for those of us with back injuries) and pedaled away for hours glued to old movies. My weight didn't change.

Something drastic had to happen. After discussing it with my partner, I decided to get a breast reduction. I lost 3.3 lb (1.5 kg) of breast fat. That was 15 years ago. It was my most significant disruption. I now jog up to 6 miles four times a week. My back is irreparable, but my BMI stays around 22.

As I get older and my weight is relatively stable, I am more interested in maintaining my flexibility, balance, and strength. My knees need strong muscles around them to protect them, and my grip has to stay strong.[7] So, I am now focusing on core strength and balance.

Most health benefits of physical activity are noticeable after 150 minutes of moderate physical intensity per week; above that, the benefits tend to plateau out. Disrupting and combining activity can extend these benefits.[8] Use Table 5.1 to help transition between types of activity when problems arise or you plateau.

For further assistance, you may join a gym. Gyms these days provide a range of equipment that can be used to improve our cardiovascular fitness, flexibility, and strength. Like all parts of a disruptive plan, I found myself searching through a series of gyms that offered different programs for obese and overweight people. Some do offer specific programs and personal coaches for very overweight people. Unfortunately, most of the equipment in most gyms is designed for fit, healthy-weight individuals. Note that some equipment can be quite dangerous for body shapes that are a larger, such as the seats on rowing machines and stationary cycles, benches, and resistance machines. You may be most comfortable, at least to start, in strength-training or other "body-shaping" classes. Going to a gym when we are overweight can be, overall, a daunting experience. Look for a place that gives you the feeling that people appreciate and support your effort.

Some gyms can be risky places—even for healthy-weight individuals. Currently, no regulations govern the setting up and operation of these

Table 5.1 Activity Prescription

	Cardiorespiratory	Strength	Flexibility
Frequency	Build up to 3–5 days/week	Build up to 2–3 times/week	Build up to 2–3 times/week
Intensity	Start light—can't feel it	Start easy—the weights seem light	Start within your range of movement—what you normally would do in a day but compacted into an exercise period
	Move to medium—you can feel your heart beat	*Move to a little harder—you can feel your muscles ache a little the next day*	*Move to focusing on improving your balance—and with it your range of movement—e.g., abdomen-strengthening exercises*
	Attempt something strenuous at least once a week—you can feel a sweat building up	**Attempt something strenuous at least once a week—you can feel your muscles shaking uncontrollably**	**Attempt something strenuous at least once a week—a flexibility class like Pilates or Yoga**
Time	Start short—e.g., 5 min/session	Start with a small number of activities—one set of exercises/session	Start short—e.g., 5 min/session
	Build up to medium—e.g., 20 min	*Build up to medium—e.g., 2–3 sets of exercises/session*	*Build up to medium—e.g., 20 min*
	Build up over a couple of months to attempt something longer once a week—e.g., 30–50 min	**Build up over a couple of months to attempt something more strenuous—e.g., 30 min of sets/week**	**Build up over a couple of months to attempt something longer once a week—e.g., 30–50 min**
Type	Continuous use of large muscle groups—e.g., walking, swimming, jogging, cycling, interval training	Intermittent against resistance using an alternating range of muscle groups	Stretching and strengthening the core muscle groups
Equipment	Very little required, but the warmup is very important.	Usually found in gyms. Best off starting with our own body as your weight and warming up with either cardiovascular exercise or flexibility exercise. Then you can move to fixed-weight machines and finally free weights.	Very little required, but the warmup is very important.

facilities beyond those applied to any commercial business. Most gyms operate in premises where space is at a premium. To maximize the use of available space, equipment is often placed close to one another, making it difficult to move around if people have mobility problems.

Treadmill injuries are not uncommon in gyms, usually resulting from a user being thrown off the back due to a fall or to an inability to keep up with the fast speed they have set. The injuries can be severe, especially if there is contact with other equipment, people, or a wall.

If you are considering a gym, visit it and note its temperature, light, and noise levels. While there are recommendations for safe air and light in gyms, they are not widely known by users. Temperature should be maintained between 68 and 72°F, with a humidity index ≤ 60%. Otherwise, overheating can cause dizziness, nausea, and loss of consciousness, especially if you are overweight and have more difficulty tolerating hot and humid environments.

While mood lighting appears to be in vogue these days in some gyms, that too can be dangerous if our balance and flexibility are not strong. In certain areas of the gym, lighting should be much higher, for example in free weights rooms, because exercises there require careful self-observation in a mirror to ensure safe technique.

Noise level can also be distracting or annoying and can counteract all the good work we do there. Eighty-five percent of instructors believe loud music motivates high-intensity class participants, but 20% of us find it stressful. I recommend using personal headphones and music. Before we sign up to a gym as part of our disruptive activity strategy, we need to make sure our safety, not just fitness, is protected.

Or create your own "gym" at home. Today a range of relatively inexpensive equipment can be safely used at home. Stability balls can be used for strengthening core muscles and stretching. Balance boards can help to sharpen reaction times and stretch muscles. Resistance bands can be used to work muscles without using weights. A variety of machines can be rented or purchased as our fitness improves, such as elliptical trainers, stationary bikes, and the like.

A wide range of gadgets are available to help us monitor how we are doing in our achievements. Many of them focus on one particular area of improvement. Pedometers measure steps taken and distances covered, and some pedometers can even translate these steps into calories. A watch-like device called a Fitbit—and a range of other similar devices—record your calories burned, number of steps taken, mileage, staircases walked, and other programmable aspects of your activity, like the amount of sleep you got that night.

Fortunately, most phones now have a pedometer app. Every time we take a step, it is recorded on the screen of the pedometer. Many apps are programmed to dictate how we should progress using built-in formulas. It is better to choose an app that learns from us and fits with our lifestyle. When we reach our goal or plateau and we can't maintain the number of steps and/or intensity of walking, we need to disrupt the program, such as a change from walking always on the flat to including a small hill.

Walking 10,000 steps per day can lower our blood pressure and increase exercise capacity, irrespective of how fast we walk or how long it takes us. Ten thousand steps is quite a lot of steps. It is best to start with fewer steps and build up slowly; for example, with a BMI over 30, walking at a low intensity for 3,000 steps is a good start. Then set realistic increases; for instance, aim to increase the number of steps by 500 weekly until you reach 10,000.

Unfortunately, pedometers don't measure the intensity of our walking. For that we require other means of measurement, such as heart rate monitors. Exercise intensity varies from person to person. Monitoring our heart rate is probably the most convenient way to assess the level of intensity. The simplest one is taking our own pulse at the wrist, not the neck because that might lead to fainting. Some exercise equipment such as fitness watches have heart rate monitors attached or built in. A range of monitors are available and even have apps.[9]

Most monitors are designed for athletes or people engaged in intensive training. Some of them are fitted around the chest, and that positioning can be a problem for those of us whose weight is mainly around the abdomen. For people who have high blood pressure and are overweight, some of their medications are designed to control the heart rate, so challenging it too much might be dangerous. In overweight and obese people, the maximum safe heart rate is calculated by a formula: 200−half the person's age. For example, a 50-year-old woman who has a BMI of 30 should not raise her heart rate beyond 175 beats/minute (200−50/2). For a person with a BMI under 25, the maximum heart rate is 220 minus their age.

Note: It is important to talk with your doctor to devise the most appropriate and safest level of exercise.

Weight around the abdomen is an increasing problem as we age. New exercise techniques such as high-intensity interval training (HIIT) or prolonged continuous exercise training show promise in moving this fat. Sessions greater than 45 minutes can also improve body composition, cardiovascular fitness, and diabetes and blood cholesterol management. Strength training has been used by people who are already doing some exercise. Strength or resistance training promotes the development of active muscle tissue instead of storing energy as fat. Strength training can involve fixed or variable weights. It is important to consult an instructor before commencing this activity. Building up too quickly or doing too much can result in serious damage to our muscles and joints. One set of 12 repetitions of a circuit, two to three times weekly has been recommended by the U.S. Surgeon General.

The results are the same, irrespective of whether we do short bursts of high-intensity workouts or longer sessions of continuous exercise. Vigorous exercise decreases our carbohydrate stores and stimulates our appetite, so watching out for the danger period of hunger after these sessions is important. Low- to moderate-intensity activity causes the most fat burning in the longer term and will lead to the largest drop in fat storage. As we increase the length of time that we exercise, we deplete more fat stores. Low- to moderate-intensity activities are more likely to be maintained in the long term than vigorous activities. For those of us with other health problems such as arthritis or heart disease, it is better to choose a regimen that is the least punishing on our joints or heart.[10]

Each of us needs to develop our own physical journey that matches our genetics, body shape, home circumstances, and work environments, all of which change through the phases of our lives. For example, we might do more general, structured, and externally organized exercise in primary and secondary school and more tailored exercise in our older years.

Diet and Physical Activity

The combined effect of diet and physical activity really works to disrupt weight in the short term. It takes between 16 weeks and one year to see changes.[11]

The amount of energy we use up in physical activity changes according to our weight and size. It is like trying to accelerate a large car versus a small one: There is more of the body to shift. For every minute of activity, Table 5.2 shows the calories burned (according to body weight).

Whatever physical activity we chose, it is important to start well within our limitations. If you are not very active, add 5 minutes of dedicated physical activity to your day,

The types of exercise we do can cause different changes in our body. Low- to moderate-intensity activity causes the most fat burning.

Without adding something beyond diet, most of us put weight back on within one to two years.

Table 5.2   Level and Type of Activity

	71 kg (156 lb)	80 kg (176 lb)	92 kg (203 lb)	98 kg (216 lb)
Low				
Sitting	1.5	1.7	1.9	2.1
Standing still	1.8	2.0	2.3	2.5
Shopping/cleaning	4.4	5.0	5.7	6.1
Cycling—slow	4.5	5.1	5.9	6.3
Walking—slow	5.7	6.4	7.4	7.8
Moderate				
Mowing lawn	7.6	9.0	10.3	11.0
Weight training	8.2	9.3	10.6	11.4
Walking—fast	8.5	9.6	11.0	11.7
Swimming—slow	9.1	9.8	11.8	12.5
Running—slow	9.2	10.9	12.5	13.3
Vigorous				
Digging in garden	10.3	11.6	13.3	14.2
Swimming—fast	11.1	12.5	14.4	15.3
Running—fast	13.7	15.4	17.8	18.9

Note: The calories expended in each of these activities may come from muscle or fat depending on our level of physical activity, fat stores, and fitness level, including muscle bulk.

every day. This is a great beginning. All the physical activity does not have to be done at once. You can add bits and pieces during the day to make up your goal. Patience is essential in the early stages. When we start disrupting our old patterns of weight loss and physical activity, the physical activity may not be as effective as a diet in achieving our weight-loss goals. However, half to one hour of physical activity three times a week can increase the effect of a diet by about 2 kg over six months. Without adding something beyond diet, most people put weight back on within one to two years.

It is important to remember that weighing ourselves may not always tell us how we are doing. Regular exercise will tone up our muscles and may even increase them in size, and muscle weighs more than fat. The benefits of our increased activity schedule may not show on the scales. The way

Table 5.3 Strategies for Overcoming the Freezers

Freezer	Thaw
I just don't have time.	Think about your total daily activity as a number of very short activities—"Tweetercises." Take a few 5- to 10-minute walks on the way to work or at lunchtime. Park a little farther away from the workplace.
The weather is too bad, too cold, or too hot.	Walk inside the mall. Walk up and down the escalators. Find an exercise video on YouTube.
I have to eat out a lot.	Plan physical activities, not meals, with friends and colleagues.
I have to travel a lot.	Walk in terminals rather than using the moving footways. Stay in hotels with gyms and use them.
I get tired when I exercise.	Good; you should. However, remind yourself that fitness will give you more energy.
I mean to do something, but I forget or can't get organized.	Place a physical activity "appointment" with yourself in your diary every day. Keep a gym bag or walking shoes in your car or at work. Join a local walking group.
This is boring.	Disrupt. Stop your current activities and try something new. Ask your friends what they are doing, and try it out.

clothes fit (looser) around your stomach and how we feel (more energetic, fitter) may be a better indication of how we are achieving our goals.

When we reach a plateau, it is important to disrupt our activities in a safe and planned way. (Table 5.1 summarizes how we can move safely between the different types of physical activity to gain cardiorespiratory fitness, strength, and flexibility.) When we plateau or lose motivation, it is important to identify our personal blocks. Table 5.3 sets out a number of common physical activity blocks in our thinking, which I have called "freezers," and with each of them I have given some suggestions on how to "thaw" them out. See how many you identify with, and even add some and then review the strategies I have suggested or write your own.

Everyone can do something; we only need to remember a few guiding principles:

1. Always know that you can do more than you thought possible.
2. Start with something you like or could like.

3. Small changes can make big changes over time.
4. Build in some non-negotiable components.
5. Remember the great feel-good effect you will get at the end.
6. Think about physical activity as healthy, not weight-reducing.
7. Listen to your body, and work within your comfort zone and at your own pace, trying not to compete with others.
8. When you plateau, disrupt . . . disrupt . . . disrupt . . .

Notes

1. http://www.sciencedirect.com/science/article/pii/S002604951630124X
2. http://journal.frontiersin.org/article/10.3389/fendo.2016.00065/full
3. http://digitalcommons.wku.edu/cgi/viewcontent.cgi?article=1895&context=ijes&sei-redir=1&referer=https%3A%2F%2Fscholar.google.co.uk%2Fscholar%3Fstart%3D50%26q%3Dreview%2Bintroducing%2B%2522physical%2Bactivity%2522%26hl%3Den%26as_sdt%3D0%2C5%26as_ylo%3D2017#search=%22review%20introducing%20physical%20activity%22
4. https://www.ncbi.nlm.nih.gov/pmc/articles/PMC1424733
5. http://www.sciencedirect.com/science/article/pii/S2090506815001050
6. https://www.researchgate.net/profile/Ray_Marks/publication/305336562_Knee_Osteoarthritis_Obesity_and_Exercise_Therapy-A_Complex_Issue/links/57c4901308ae9b0c824c26c5.pdf
7. http://onlinelibrary.wiley.com/doi/10.1111/obr.12422/full
8. http://midus.wisc.edu/findings/pdfs/1616.pdf
9. http://www.livescience.com/49653-best-heart-rate-monitor-apps.html
10. https://www.hindawi.com/journals/jdr/2017/5071740/abs
11. https://www.ncbi.nlm.nih.gov/books/NBK62231

CHAPTER SIX

Customizing Our Approach

We all have our preferred ways of doing things and interacting with others. The purpose of this chapter is to help us understand our most comfortable way of doing things so that we can increase our effectiveness in disrupting weight in the long term.

Our behavior is changeable depending on the environment we are in, the activity we are doing, and the people we are with; for example, how we behave at work is different from how we might behave as a parent. Behavior can also change over time as we learn new ways of operating and gain confidence. In this chapter, we will be looking at our behaviors related to weight reduction and maintenance and how we can maximize them to ensure a lifetime of healthy weight.

For at least two decades, I have been using a modified questionnaire to help the people I work with to identify the strategies that will work best for them.[1] Again, it's like buying a pair of shoes. They look alright and are even our usual size, but some pairs are still uncomfortable. We have hope that they will be alright, and we buy them. Then they sit in our wardrobe, unworn, gathering dust, and reminding us every time we open the door that we made a mistake. They are just like the dieting books with diets that looked good for a time and now sit on the shelf or the computer programs and apps that promised weight loss, delivered for only a short period of time, and now blink at us from our computers and phones.

It is an important lesson to learn. We have to match the kind of strategies we are going use with what we feel most comfortable trying.[2] Of course, losing weight won't be comfortable in the beginning, but we can make it as easy as possible with the right choices. The questionnaire in Table 6.1 will help identify how we get to our preferred behavioral style when it

Table 6.1 Disruptive Weight Questionnaire

Director	Influencer	Team member	Academic
1. Bold _____	Enthusiastic _____	Good-natured _____	Conscientious _____
2. Daring _____	Talkative _____	Easygoing _____	Logical _____
3. Vigorous _____	Outgoing _____	Agreeable _____	Careful _____
4. Strong-willed _____	Charming _____	Sympathetic _____	Tactful _____
5. Pioneering _____	Talkative _____	Gentle _____	Well disciplined _____
6. Competitive _____	Sociable _____	Even-tempered _____	Thorough _____
7. Restless _____	Sociable _____	Considerate _____	Controlled _____
8. Direct _____	High-spirited _____	Kind _____	Reserved _____
9. Vigorous _____	Expressive _____	Amiable _____	Accurate _____
10. Dominant _____	Sociable _____	Easy going _____	Controlled _____
Scores for each column:	_____	_____	_____

Highest score _____   Second highest score _____

comes to losing weight. It contains 10 lines, each containing four statements. In each line of statements, rank each adjective as to how it most accurately describes how we behave when trying to lose weight:

4 points to the word that best describes you

3 points to the word that is like you

2 points to the word that is a bit like you

1 point to the word that least describes you

Do not spend a long time thinking about your answers.

Your highest score best describes your most comfortable approach to losing weight. Your second highest comes next. We will now look at how these styles can help you chose which strategies you can use and when.

Director

If you scored highest in the first column (Director), you are most comfortable choosing a style of losing weight that you can direct. You will gravitate to programs that you can control yourself and that are fast and simple and achieve rapid results. You need to make sure that you change your programs often because you like the fast pace. You also need to steer away from any activities that involve a lot of group work because you like to be quite independent when you think of losing weight. A low-fat diet might be good for you to start with because it is easy to count fat, and the lists of foods you need to avoid are short. Similarly, an exercise program that you can download onto your phone and that changes frequently would keep you motivated. Stay away from group counseling sessions or long one-on-one sessions. You are very likely to get demotivated.

Bassey

Recall the case of Bassey in Chapter 2. Bassey is obese and over 6′ tall. He has lost up to 28.5 kg (63 lb) several times but has put it back on again within the space of a year. When he loses it, he can exercise and frequently completes 10-km (6-mile) fun runs. He and his partner came around for dinner. His partner had told me beforehand that this month they were on diets and so they weren't drinking alcohol. I made a low-fat seafood bisque with rice. Bassey put a small amount of food on his plate and then asked me if there was any bread. I was surprised that he asked for bread given they were on a diet. In any case, I didn't have any bread. Bassey looked disappointed. Clearly he wanted some bread to dunk into the bisque. I wasn't sure what to do about dessert as I hadn't made anything because they said they were on a diet. I had some leftover fruit cake and placed it on a plate with some fruit for dessert. I cut the cake into three medium-sized pieces and left the apples and banana whole. Bassey cut one piece of the fruit cake into three smaller sections, and we all took one of the small pieces. By the time they left the dining table, all the remaining pieces of cake had gone into Bassey's mouth—and none of the fruit was touched.

Later that the evening, Bassey asked me how this book was going (I was nearly finished with the first draft) and what was going to make this book stand out from all the others in the bookshops and on the Web sites. I told him it was a simple message: Weight maintenance is a lifelong process of disrupting unhelpful activities and processes that are no longer effective. Relapses are common and should not make us ashamed or give up. We should just learn from them and act differently. Bassey looked interested and asked me how it would work with him. I asked him fill out the questionnaire. He came up as a weight Director.

The most important thing for Bassey was to stop responding to his partner's attempts to put him on a diet and abandon crash dieting. Those strategies weren't working long term for him. He needed to try a series of task-focused elimination techniques that he directed and owned for himself. The first one was food elimination. I made him list his top 10 favorite foods in descending order of preference, described earlier in this book. What I was seeking to do was to help him identify something he liked that he could eliminate forever.

Over time, with each elimination success, we can stop controlling what we eat and enjoy what we like that is healthy. It is a series of short-term processes. Bassey's top five favorite foods now change frequently because he wants to keep disrupting his body while still having the food and drink he likes. He continues to maintain his weight loss.

Influencer

If you scored highest in the second column (Influencer), you are most comfortable choosing a style of losing weight that is social and fast paced. You will enjoy programs where you are participating in a group and where you can express your thoughts and feelings. You are not very good with detailed work, so steer away from programs that require a lot of attention, like calorie-controlled diets. Groups such as Weight Watchers might be good for you. Similarly, a local community center or gym with a variety of classes would be the best way to keep you motivated to exercise. Stay away from rigid programs that require regular follow-up because you will only feel guilty when you inevitably miss some sessions.

Cal

After Cal retired, he stopped going to the gym with his work colleagues, and no one invited him on the fun runs or bicycle tours anymore. He stayed at home most days, and his weight continued to gradually increase. Within nine months, he weighed more than 130 kg (300 lb). His lifestyle had become quite relaxed, now that he no longer had to travel to work every day, attend exercise classes with his colleagues, and watch his diet. He had fallen into an armchair and virtually stayed there all winter. Three months later, when his knees started aching, he went to a local doctor and was diagnosed with type 2 diabetes. He then came to me to discuss how to disrupt the pattern he had gotten himself into. Cal wanted to lose half his weight in a year, but we set a more realistic goal of approximately 60 lb during the next year. Together, we planned a get-out-of-the-house weight-loss program. Every month, he had to add something new to do—preferably in a group situation. The first trio of strategies was a local diabetic patients group, a university of the third-age yoga class, and a membership with the local bowling club. Then Cal decided he liked these new ideas and joined a healthy cooking class, went on healthy retreats, and decided to do a course to become a disability fitness instructor. Within two years, he had lost 47 kg (105 lb) and was worried that he might put it back on as he was too tired from everything he was doing to give much attention to his wife, and she was bored with all the "restrictions." These support activities helped Cal achieve his goal but could not be sustained until his body reset itself in a way that let him adjust to a life in which his wife could participate. We discussed disruption, and he agreed to try a long-term program that engaged his wife. Cal bought his wife a 10-year desk planner so that their combined retirement occupation could be disruptive weight maintenance.

Team Member

If you scored highest in the third column (Team Member), you are most comfortable choosing a style of losing weight that focuses on groups of people and that is not rushed. You prefer participating in a group that is agreeable, where you don't have to say very much, and the decisions are made for you keeping in mind not only yourself but also other people you care about. An organized group that you could attend with like-minded people would suit you the best. Perhaps a weight-loss group of parents from your children's school might be a good place to start. Similarly, an exercise program that fits in with the needs of the others—such as a dog walking group—would suit you best. You have a tendency to get comfortable with one type of program and so may stay too long in it—past when it still works for you—sometimes because you don't want to disappoint your friends. It is a good idea to remember that your losing weight is also important to those around you whom you care about, so changing programs might be necessary to achieve your long-term goals.

Sista

Sista was always a poor eater. When her mom used to pick her up from day care after work, Sista would still be sitting in front of a plate of cold boiled spinach from lunchtime. When Sista married and had her sons, she did what every money-conscious mother would do: She wouldn't let the boys' leftovers go to waste. The half-eaten sandwiches would be eaten either by herself or her husband. Everybody in their community did it. The boys were little, and she was very active running around after them. She never noticed the weight slowly creeping up around her waist and bottom.

When her mother got sick with cancer, Sista would sit all day with her. Her mother thought that if she kept eating, it meant that she was winning the fight against the cancer. Sista would eat with her mother, then go home and eat with the family. When her mother eventually died, Sista was huge and depressed, and food was even more important as a comfort and shared memory of her time with her mother at the end. Her menopause didn't help either as her bra size increased to a 42GGG.

Sista had never tried dieting. She said she didn't care. Her husband liked her as she was. It was only when they had to move to a different house because her knees hurt too much climbing stairs that she came to see me for a referral to an orthopedic surgeon in order to get her knees replaced. The surgeon told her they weren't that bad but scheduled the surgery anyway. Sista decided that her family couldn't do without her while she got better, and I didn't see her for a year.

When she came to see me again, her husband had been diagnosed with diabetes and they were both going to a family weight-loss group run by her cousin who was a dietician. Since starting, Sista had lost 10 kg (22 lb). Now everyone in the group had plateaued and was going to see their doctors about weight-loss surgery. Sista wanted me to refer her to a bariatric surgeon for gastric banding because she couldn't lose any more weight. Her knees were a little better, and her blood pressure and cholesterol were okay.

She said the whole family was getting used to the new way of eating. Sista and I talked about her successes using peer support and family pressure. She agreed that they were great motivators and would continue to be.

Academic

If you scored highest in the fourth column (Academic), you are most comfortable choosing a style of losing weight that focuses on all the available evidence and research you can find. You will like to take your time and weigh up everything you see, read, and hear before making a decision. Doing all this may take you a long time to start. This book has a lot of reliable references for you to read, which should give you a place to start. Because of your fastidious nature, any program that provides a lot of detail will work for you, for example calorie counting, food composition analysis, or structured complex exercise programs. You may find that groups do not look at the evidence in enough detail for you, so they may frustrate and demotivate you. You may benefit from some serious discussion with a range of health professionals in order to develop a long-term set of strategies from the outset.

Dolly

Dolly is a director of nursing. I first met Dolly when we were doing some research together. We talked on the phone and skyped quite often. It was only when I met her in person that I saw how obese she really was. She managed to cover up her huge upper arms with black tops and was always sitting down when we turned the cameras on. She had a phobia of public speaking because people would see how large she was. She had missed out on several jobs at the interview because of her size.

She was morbidly obese, and her long-term partner Jaye was even larger. She had no cardiovascular or orthopedic problems, nor was she diabetic. She was what some people like to call the "healthy obese person."

Years later, I was working with her in her office on a paper when she offered to go to the café and bring back some lunch. Some 20 minutes later, she came back with two veggie wraps (each one cut in half, and each half large enough for one person), a large pasta salad (from a different café), and two fruit smoothies. "All very healthy," she said, as she knew I was a vegetarian. I told Dolly that I didn't like pasta anymore (it had been off my top 10 list for years), so perhaps she could take it home.

Clearly, Dolly had a problem with portion size. We discussed my belief in disruptive processes, and I gave her a number of articles to read. She decided that because she had no medical conditions, a lack of physical fitness was her main problem. After reviewing the literature thoroughly, she decided to get an exercise program for her gaming console.

In the beginning, we are very motivated and have a strong commitment to lose weight by whatever first disruptive strategy we have chosen, be it dieting or another approach. We can hear ourselves saying, "This time I really want to lose weight." But in the back of our minds, we know we haven't got many skills to draw on. We are "unconsciously incompetent"— we don't know what we don't know. In this stage, we need to be thinking whether we have clear enough goals. How much weight do we realistically aim to lose in the first six months? Which initial strategy best fits our behavioral style? A rigid diet? A community group? We might also need someone to show us what to do, like counting fat grams per day, or practicing mindfulness, or hiring a therapist.

Within a month of daily exercises, Dolly developed bursitis in her hip, which through a series of complications, led to an unstable hip replacement. Dolly lost her confidence and motivation. Exercise was clearly the wrong primary strategy for her. Dolly's problem was more complex and included behavioral elements. She decided to consult a center that gave a fully integrated bariatric surgery approach—with counselors, diet plans, exercise programs, and physiotherapy.

Inevitably, disappointments will occur, especially if the tasks we have set ourselves are too ambitious or if, despite what we are doing, the weight is not coming off at a rate that gives us reassurance that we are doing the right things. We might start thinking that we can never lose weight and that the process in the long term is not as easy as it looks in this book. At that point, we are becoming consciously incompetent—we now are starting to know that we need more skills and disruptive thinking to continue on the disruptive weight path. Our commitment may wane, and we may even think of giving up. It is in this phase that our disruptive thinking and actions are most important. It important here to have enough strategies at hand to change direction again if we fail. Strong support from those around is also important. Friends, clinicians, and colleagues should be recruited to be available in this phase.

After much discussion, Dolly had a gastric band inserted, which helped her lose 10% body weight and let her retrain her intake with respect to appropriate portion size. Then it became dislodged. She had it removed and, at the same time, had a gastric sleeve operation, which from the emerging evidence was more suitable to her problems. She has lost another 10% of body weight.

With persistence and support, each of us can overcome our disappointments and lapses and reach a place where we feel competent in our ability to continue weight management.

Learning to Master Long-Term Weight Disruption

Making change permanent is easier than we think. By assessing how we are doing along the way to reach specific weight-loss goals, we make what seems a daunting task manageable. The model I have used for years is based on the premise that whenever we learn to do something new, we go through a series of learning stages. At each stage, we need to assess what we need to make it to the next stage. Sometimes we can do it on our own; other times, we might need help. When we learn a new task, we use two of our attributes. One is our competence, or the level of knowledge and skill we have to perform the task. In the beginning, this is always low. The other is our commitment, or the degree of motivation we possess to master the task and the confidence that we can. This varies along the process, but if we aren't motivated in the beginning, we will never succeed. The fact that you are reading this book shows a certain level of motivation, which is a good start. Competence and commitment fluctuate, but we go through four phases on the way. We start as an enthusiastic beginner and work our way through disenchantment until we become capable and, finally, self-reliant.

Notes

1. Supervising research students in primary health care using a leadership model. Saltman D, O'Dea N, https://www.ncbi.nlm.nih.gov/pubmed/15227871

2. Weight management information sheets. Saltman DC, O'Dea NA. *AFP.* 2000, 29 (4), 307, 313, 319, 327, 333.

CHAPTER SEVEN

Distortion and Disruption

Body distortions can sometimes hinder a successful weight disruption program. Body image is the way our minds conceive a mental picture of the size, shape, and form of our bodies.[1] It has two components: the way we perceive our body size and how satisfied we are with it. When we're obese or overweight, we have a higher level of body distortion and dissatisfaction as compared to normal-weight people, and the extent of our distortion increases with our size. In females, this degree of distortion usually correlates with a patient's BMI status. Body dissatisfaction affects both females and males, although it is more common in women. In females, dissatisfaction tends to be directed toward being larger than desired, while in males the focus is on insufficient muscularity.

Tiffany

Tiffany knows when she has put on too much weight by how many of her bones she can get feel through her skin. She especially likes to check her hip bones after eating and squeeze the fat on her abdomen between her fingers every morning when she wakes up. Although she can be temporarily reassured when she feels her hip bones, doing so is a problem because it remains an issue in her daily life and doesn't let her focus on other things. She never looks in the mirror beyond putting on her makeup because she is ashamed of what she sees.

In the high school gym changing rooms, all the girls compare themselves in the mirrors to one another. Tiffany is quite developed for her age, and she is very proud of her breasts, especially because all the boys like looking at her. It is the rest of her body that she despises, so she makes shaming comparisons with the other girls and with models in magazines. She never goes near mirrors.

Mirrors have the potential to provide misleading but highly acceptable information, and it is likely that they play an important role in maintaining our body dissatisfaction. As with other forms of body checking, what we find to be true and what we believe to be true depends on what we look at and how. Tiffany had learned the hard way that detailed scrutiny, especially of her perceived defects, only magnified her flaws in her mind and, she believed, showed them off to the other girls.

Tiffany was right that mirrors are useful for applying makeup, arranging hair, or, for men, shaving. For Tiffany to move beyond that, she had to disrupt the way she used mirrors. First, she had to just look at herself in the mirror. It didn't initially matter how quickly she looked. Gradually, she increased her time looking at herself until the anxiety she felt disappeared. The most important challenge was to keep looking until the anxiety or distress diminished. She agreed that the final goal was to look at herself in a full-length mirror wearing underwear.

Early on, we did a reality test related to the feelings she had in the school gym changing room. I asked:

> What do the girls in the gym and the models in the media typically look like? What has to be done to touch up a model before she has her photo taken? What sort of manipulation is done after the photo is taken? What message is the advertiser sending you when the product is presented alongside an ideal image of this model in a successful situation?

We discussed what she could do, on a continuing basis, to disrupt the unrealistic views of others and the negative views of herself. First, she had to stop looking "upward," that is, at the features of the girls and models who she thought had desirable qualities such as small thighs and waists, and compare herself to other girls who had less desirable qualities such as bad acne or bigger thighs than her. In other words, she needed to widen her perspective to see her "better" physical traits. Then she had to work through an agreed list of the attributes that she looked up to and those she looked down on, and she had to switch one from one list to the other every time she felt anxious about seeing herself in the mirror or other girls in the changing rooms.

Sometimes, we have beliefs that are way off the truth mark and that can sabotage our weight-loss quest unless they are removed. My patient, Duane, offered an example. "Even though I trust the nutritionist that you recommended, I still believe that yogurt will make me fat," Duane explained. "He keeps telling me that it's all about portion control and that no one food group can make a person fat. I know he is right, because my wife reads everything she can find, and she agrees with him. But . . . ."

Portion control is, in fact, important, and the lack of it is one of the main culprits keeping us fat. Big portions mean more calories, of course. And sometimes aren't so easy to notice. With any large-size portion of food, such as a large bag of popcorn, a lot of calories can be eaten before we notice any change in the contents of the bag. Even if we look at the packet beforehand to gauge how calorie-rich it is, we can be deceived. Labels on food packaging can be unhelpful; for example, unrealistically small serving sizes are used on food packages to suggest that there are more servings in the package and that the calorie content is not excessive.[2] In restaurants, jumbo-sized portions are over 200% larger than regular portions. Even at home, portion size can be a problem not of our own making. Bowls and plates are one-third larger than they were in 1960.[3]

As portions have grown over the years, so have our overweight issues. Table 7.1 present general examples, along with estimates of size and caloric changes, as well as how long we have to be active to burn up those extra calories.

Portion size is more of an issue for men than for women. Some strategies that Duane was taught to help him disrupt his problems with portions include repackaging purchased foods into smaller units; making sure always to eat from a plate, not a package; after repacking in small units, storing bulk foods away from direct vision or, better yet, freezing them; and saving part of each meal for another time. We still had to confront the problems that his wife experienced in preparing the portions, such as the extra washing up of measuring equipment, such as scales, and hot foods, such as cooked pasta, getting cold while being measured, but the approach worked for Duane. Physically, at least.

"Although I am nearing my goal weight, I still feel fat," he said.

Quite often, we can change our behaviors—and our bodies—but our thought patterns lag behind. I explained that "feeling fat" is not the same as being fat. Our feelings about and our memories of our earlier, bigger bodies tend to fluctuate markedly from day to day and even within the day. They are not the same as being unhappy about our current body shape. This is an example of a time when mindfulness training—living in the moment—may be useful. It is something we can all do—stay focused on the now and on what we have achieved.

Table 7.1   Portion Distortion*

Bagel

Twenty years ago, a 3-in. diameter bagel contained 140 calories.

Today, bagels are generally bigger, with a 6-in. diameter and 350 calories.

To lose that extra 210 calories, we would have to do 50 minutes of moderate strenuous activity, such as raking leaves.

Cheeseburger

Twenty years ago, a cheeseburger was 330 calories at about 3 oz.

Today, it is 590 calories at about 5 oz.

Losing those extra 260 calories requires 90 minutes of moderate strenuous activity, for example lifting small weights.

Spaghetti and meatballs

Twenty years ago, 1 c of spaghetti, sauce, and three meatballs were about 500 calories.

Today, we often eat two cups of spaghetti, sauce, and three meatballs at 1,000 calories.

Losing those extra 500 calories requires 2.5 hours of moderate activity, for example active house cleaning.

French fries

Twenty years ago, a serving (2.5 oz) of French fries contained 200 calories.

Today, a serving (6.5 oz) of French fries contains 600 calories.

Losing those extra 400 calories requires an hour of low-impact physical activity like walking.

Soda

Twenty years ago, a bottle of soda (6.5 oz) contained 85 calories.

Today, an average bottle of soda (20 oz) contains 250 calories.

Losing those extra 165 calories requires 30 minutes of moderate physical activity, for example gardening.

Turkey sandwich

Twenty years ago, a turkey sandwich contained 300 calories.

Today, a turkey sandwich contains 800 calories.

Losing those extra 500 calories requires 1.5 hours of strenuous physical activity, for example bike riding.

*Approximate estimates only.

Notes

1. http://onlinelibrary.wiley.com/doi/10.1038/oby.2009.418/full
2. https://ijbnpa.biomedcentral.com/articles/10.1186/1479-5868-6-58
3. http://www.smallplatemovement.org/doc/big_portions.pdf

CHAPTER EIGHT

Binge Eating: A Warning about the Destructive Weight Disruption

Binge eating and obesity often go together. And when they do, we have two major problems, not one, to manage. Whereas obesity is largely a problem of uncontrolled, excessive eating, binge eating has the additional problem that each uncontrolled meal is matched with an equally uncontrolled excessive output. When we binge, we eat more than most people would and in a short period of time, and we can't control ourselves. Remorseful and guilty, we follow up a binge with a purging of calories, such as by vomiting, the overuse of laxatives or diuretics, enemas, fasting, or excessive exercise.[1]

> *Binge eating is not a beneficial disruptive weight management action.*

Aisha

Aisha is a 36-year-old, unmarried personnel manager, who lives at home with her family. She is 5'3" tall and weighs 132 kg (291 lb), giving her a BMI of nearly 40. She said she put on 80 lb over the last year because her boyfriend left her. Work was going okay, but she was not dating anyone.

She had been obese and a binge eater since she was 10 years old. She believes she was singled out as the "chubby" daughter and was treated differently from her three older siblings (brothers and sisters) at meal-times. Her parents had always been worried about her weight, and they enrolled her in her first weight-loss program at the age of 12. That is also when she recalls her first episode of binge eating. For the next 25 years, she cycled through periods of weight loss of between 20 and 80 lb, usually by participating in weight-loss programs or popular diets, and then she would regain the weight in periods of uncontrolled binge eating. Aisha's weight was stable for no more than six months and then was either going up or down.

Aisha's story is typical of many of us who are have been led to believe that one strategy, if we stick to it, will keep the weight off for life. The dangerous reality is that Aisha's binge eating is an example of disruptive weight management that is clearly not a beneficial type. What Aisha needed to do was replace the binge disruptions each time she felt drawn to them with something more helpful to keeping weight off, rather than putting more on. Instead of a demoralizing cycle of weight loss and regain, Aisha had to make her disruptions into something far more positive. Here are snippets from the consultations when we met:

Me: How has bulimia helped you?

Aisha: I don't know. No one has ever asked me that before. Everyone just tells me how dangerous it is.

Me: Well, I think if we work together so you can understand the process of how and why you disrupt your weight in unhelpful ways and what parts of the disruption work for you, we might be able to change your disruptions from unhealthy to helpful . . . and develop a way forward that is manageable for the rest of your life.

Aisha: Well, now I get to eat whatever I want and know that I can get rid of it anytime I choose. And when I have a bad day, bingeing takes over, and while I am bingeing, I forget what is upsetting me.

Me: So bingeing helps you feel less scared about putting on weight and also lets you feel okay about eating anything you want when you need to.

Aisha: Yes, but it doesn't always work. I am obsessed with food. All I ever think about is what I've eaten, what I shouldn't eat, and what I'm going to eat. It's hard to concentrate on anything else. And I feel really sick after I binge and purge. Often, when I do it at night, I feel too feel weak and dizzy to brush my teeth and now the dentist says my teeth are rotting away.

Me: I'm glad you came, and I know we can find a better way forward.

. . .

Me: What other things do you wish you could concentrate on instead of thinking about food?

Aisha: Well, I'd like to have children soon; before I get too old, and I don't think I can get another partner. I think my last one left me because I got too fat.

Me: So you have a lot of things going on. There is the binge eating, which helps calm you when you are upset, and the purging after lets you worry less about gaining weight. But you still are putting on weight, and these negative disruptive cycles make it hard for you to concentrate on other things in your life and takes a lot of your time away from the other things you value.

Aisha's high levels of preoccupation with thoughts of food and weight came from the way issues related to food and eating were central in her family's thoughts and actions. Much of her interaction with her family members focused on food, eating, or weight gain. The family's reliance on one type of weight management concept, in this case, commercial weight-loss programs, only made Aisha feel worse when she inevitably failed.

> *Despite all our hopes, there is no one single strategy for weight maintenance that works forever.*

Despite all our hopes, there is no one single strategy for weight maintenance that works lifelong.

We talked about narrowing Aisha's focus to the here and now and about recognizing that she has well established skills to cease doing something—especially when it isn't working for her—whether it is bingeing, purging, or dieting. She recognized, though, that trying anything new felt difficult because of her negative associations from the past.

Aisha's Personalized Disruption

Aisha was always successful in the initial phases of a weight reduction program, so we discussed which ones might work again for her in the beginning. She made a list of all the programs she had signed up for and how long she had lasted in each of them. In total, she had been on at least 10 programs, and the average time she lasted in each was seven months. She then rated the top three that worked best (not necessarily the longest) and why. The three that she picked had these things in common: They were good value for money; the diets were manageable within the limitations of what she could get locally and what she was prepared to eat; and she didn't feel guilty when she stopped them.

She then had to complete some homework, which was to search the Internet to find any new programs that matched what worked for her before. Together, we made a list of promising programs and what signals she should look for to help her work out whether to change from one program to another—always based on the failure signals she recognized, such as missing meetings, substituting foods, occasional overeating, and weight plateauing.

We also had to deal with Aisha's family. Families who have to deal with long-term weight problems in their children often engage in predictable, guilt-inducing and destructive behaviors. In Aisha's case, her mother was usually the one who took on the role of peacemaker when Aisha's father started calling Aisha fat. Differences of opinion would appear and split the family. Some family members would "side" with the peacemaking activities, trying to not to make things worse. Other family members, usually her brothers, would say nothing and distance themselves to avoid dealing with the problem. Aisha would feel not only fat but also guilty about the extra attention given to her, as well as being ashamed about the way some of her family ignored her. When her sisters eventually tried to help, often it was too late. Aisha felt that the extra attention was controlling rather than caring.

Table 8.1   Segment from Aisha's Nighttime Plan

Recognize the Situation and the Emotions	Disruptive Response
What happened that evening when I felt the urge to eat or was in an upsetting situation? How did I feel (anxious, sad, angry)?	What could I do instead?
Example:	**I could have:**
6 p.m.: I bought 2 packets of my favorite cookies at the register while buying some painkillers for my period pain, and I was scared I would eat them during the night. So I ate both of them while cleaning up after dinner, since I was still hungry.	Gone to another shop that didn't have tempting things at the checkout counter. Bought something healthier and convinced myself I would like it more. Asked someone in the family to hold the cookies for me. Eaten enough during my meals and snacks in the day, so that I would be better able to control my eating during the night. Thrown the cookies away.

Aisha's family described a range of approaches they had to helping Aisha lose weight, but they admitted that, over time, all their strategies decreased in effectiveness and led to less and less commitment from the family to help Aisha. Clearly, some families, not just individuals, need to practice approach disruption. Aisha's parents said they felt helpless and despaired for Aisha. They knew that winning the battle at the dinner table did not change Aisha's behavior later. Aisha had to come up with her own night-time plan (see Table 8.1). Commitment from her family not to continue on their guilt-inducing ways was the best Aisha could seek.

Note

1. http://www.sciencedirect.com/science/article/pii/S0193953X05702288

CHAPTER NINE

Learning to Live without Obesity

The benefits of maintaining healthy weight in the long term are many. Our hearts are in better shape—both the physical and the emotional one.[1] Even a 10% weight loss can have a major effect on lowering our blood pressure.[2] We are more mobile and walk better.[3] We sleep better.[4] We use 11% less medications, go to hospital 10% less, and lower our health care costs by $600 per year.[5] For those of us who undergo bariatric surgery, our risks of heart attacks and strokes are halved.[6]

Many activities of daily living also change once we disrupt the weight that held us hostage. Some of these events can be pleasurable, such as finding healthy food and physical activity pleasurable and not a chore or not having to worry about finding a seat large enough at a concert or asking for a seat belt extender in an airplane. We find new activities that we could not get involved in before, from walking around fairgrounds to strolling the streets and meeting new or greeting old neighbors.

Jaye

Jaye is 43 and has managed to keep her BMI at 57.3 lb/m^2 (26 kg/m^2) for eight years now. She has spent much of her life focused on losing weight, treating her body as the enemy, or trying to ignore it. She came to see me because she was worried about small things that now caught her attention, such as the small weight gain (a few pounds) that she could not prevent in the depths of winter and the monthly weight changes around her menses. These small changes were manageable but tended to preoccupy her thoughts.

Successfully disrupting our heavy actions and thoughts for the longer term can seem like the ultimate goal. Yet when this is achieved, finding a way forward in life can be difficult.[7] Jaye had no idea what to do with herself now that she had successfully disrupted those destructive patterns. Learning to reenter the world, especially one so focused on obesity, is not always easy. We are programmed when we are young regarding how we look, and this hardwiring is difficult to shift, even if we recognize that what we think about ourselves now might be inaccurate and unfair. Seeing ourselves as obese is familiar and has a kind of perverse comfort, even though we may no longer be overweight.

Also, those who are close to us may not be able to conquer their thoughts about us. When Jaye started wearing her new clothes that were better contoured to her slimmed-down body, her husband Cal started calling her "skinny." She didn't mind being called "fat," and even thought it a lot about herself and her overweight friends, but she really didn't like being called "skinny." It made her wonder what her husband was really thinking and whether he really didn't support all her efforts to lose weight.

When we all got together, Cal admitted that he was threatened by Jaye's ultimate success in losing weight. While she was in the process of losing weight, he felt that they were in it together. Now that she had achieved a healthy weight, he didn't know what they had to share anymore, and he was worried that she would leave him. He missed the connection they had in thinking about disrupting what they ate long term. Jaye was a now a different person from the one he married. Sometimes he thought she was like a model in a magazine, even distant and unapproachable. At those times, he called her "skinny."

Jaye and Cal needed to work together on new life challenges. When they thought about it, a lot of their friends were overweight and still struggling to attain a healthy weight long term. Some of them asked for advice. Others were jealous of Jaye's success and even tried to sabotage her efforts; for example, when they all went out to dinner, they would make unhealthy suggestions about what she should choose to eat and place food on her plate. They couldn't believe that a woman who had devoured big burgers and gobs of fries could really now like salads.

Disrupting her lifelong weight problem had given Jaye the confidence to consider other disruptions. She felt she had the opportunity to start afresh and was worried that it couldn't happen in their current circumstances. She and Cal are now considering a move to a new neighborhood or even a new city, where they can celebrate what they had achieved and look for new challenges.

Shedding the ties that bind us to people who are comfortable with seeing us overweight is difficult. It is made even more difficult when our bodies remind us of what we have lost. Looking every day at drooping, fat-depleted breasts and aprons of skin across our abdomens, upper arms, and buttocks can be harsh reminders.

Excess Skin

Our genes may affect how our skin responds to weight gain and loss. Several other factors also contribute to sagging skin after weight loss. The longer we have been overweight or obese, the looser our skin will be. The more weight we lose, the more our skin hangs. For example, with weight loss greater than 100 lb (45.4 kg), we can expect large areas of hanging skin.[8] Stretched skin loses the ability to be flexible because we lose a lot of the elastin and collagen that helps maintain our skin elasticity. Chronic sun exposure, aging, and smoking can make it worse because they also reduce collagen and elastin.

Excess skin also can be uncomfortable and interfere with our daily activities. One of the first things to do is exercise. Three-quarters of us find that loose skin prevents us from exercising. The problem may be worse for those who go to gyms. Nearly half of us will stop going because we can't stand people staring at our flapping skin. Also, for nearly half of us, excess skin folds can trap heat and moisture, which can lead to skin infections, usually fungal ones such as *Candida*.

Many creams on the market are supposed to "firm" our skin and get rid of stretch marks. Early-stage stretch marks, that is, those that are still red and haven't become white, respond to trentinoin (Retin A) gels. They cause defects in the babies of people who use them, so they cannot be used in people who are of childbearing age. Other creams, such as those containing glycolic acid, commonly called "fruit peels," can give a slight boost to skin tightness, but the effect is only temporary because the collagen and elastin that are required for long-lasting firmness cannot be absorbed through the skin. Once the stretch marks turn white, very little can be done short of surgical interventions.

Most medical or surgical treatments can be done outside hospitals. Many devices are available for tightening, including radio frequency, infrared devices, combinations, and ultrasound. The results of these techniques are mixed.[9] All skin-tightening techniques work by changing the environment under our skin—usually through heat—and causing inflammation. The collagen under our skin contracts like when we get a scar. However, the tightening is only temporary, and after the effect wears off, the skin can be more stretched.

For some of us, plastic surgery is necessary to rectify these problems. This is especially true for those of us who have had bariatric surgery. Two out of every three of those of us who have bariatric surgery choose to have body-contouring surgery to remove excess skin.[10] Specific body-contouring surgeries include abdominoplasty, commonly called "tummy tuck" (which removes skin from the abdomen); lower body lift (which removes skin from the belly, buttocks, hips, and thighs); upper body lift (which removes skin from the breasts and back); medial thigh lift (which removes skin from the inner and outer thighs); and brachioplasty, commonly known as "arm lift" (which removes skin from the upper arms). Breasts are another area where surgery can assist in rectifying skin laxity, deflation, and dropping of the breasts.[11] Multiple surgeries are usually required for the different regions.

Most body-contouring surgery is done within two years of achieving stable weight loss.[12] The procedure usually requires a hospital stay of one to four days. Recovery time at home takes between two to four weeks, and compression garments have to be worn after the surgery to keep the shape in place until the skin readjusts.[13] The surgery has some potential complications, such as bleeding, breakdown of stitches, opening of the wound, and infections. These complications are more common with larger amounts of weight loss and after gastric bypass surgery.[14]

Persistent Organic Pollutants and Fat

Our fat tissue is an organ that can store fat-soluble chemicals that are not easily metabolized and excreted from the body. When we experience rapid or major weight loss, these chemicals, called "persistent organic pollutants" (POPs), are released from our fat tissue in larger than usual amounts. POPs are mainly found in fatty animal products such as fish, meat, and milk (including breast milk). Typical examples of POPs are chlorinated compounds such as organochlorine pesticides, polychlorinated biphenyls, and dioxins. These POPs degrade slowly under normal body conditions and are primarily excreted in feces or through bile. When we have excess fat, these POPs are stored and not excreted.

As we lose weight and for some time after, the amount of POPs released into our circulation increases, and the POPs have a greater chance of reaching toxic levels in critical organs, such as the gallbladder, liver, brain, pancreas, and thyroid glands. For example, POPs can block bile secretion from the liver and cause gallstones.[15] Circulating POPs can rise by 150–400% following a 40% bodyweight loss and stay around for up to one year.[16]

Exposure to POPs has also been associated with diabetes, metabolic syndrome, alterations of thyroid function, some cancers, infertility, and other neurological, hormonal, and immunological problems.[17] POPs-related problems due to weight loss are more serious in older adults than in younger adults, probably because older people have a longer time to accumulate them and are less efficient at getting rid of them. Some evidence is also emerging that high concentrations of POPs released from fat tissue into the bloodstream during intensive weight loss could promote subsequent weight regain.[18]

Frequently changing the type of maintenance strategies we do, such as altering our rate of weight loss, can prevent the rapid release of POP-laden fat into the bloodstream.

Shedding Old Habits

Most of who successfully lose weight have spent our lives focusing on how to hide our lumps and bumps from the world. It is no wonder we have very little idea how to dress ourselves in our new body shape. Being able to fit into smaller-size clothes doesn't make shopping any simpler. In fact, the increased range of choice can make it more difficult for us. Some styles will be easier to try on but still not fit our body shape or look good. Clothing fit is often more about shape than weight, so even if we size down, many of our previous challenges, such as big hips and thighs, will stay challenging. Also, it is easy to fall into the trap of waiting to start shopping until we reach our goal weight. Waiting only leads to our staying in the wrong clothes and looking at our old self every day—not our new self. Dressing for the moment is important to confirm our new selves. In our transition phase, it helps to stay thrifty, such as tailoring clothes instead of buying new ones or getting castoffs from others in our weight management group. Shopping online can be problematic until we know what suits us and helps to build up enough confidence to go a department store to try on different sizes and designs. Or try going to a secondhand store, where the atmosphere may feel more welcoming, less judgmental.

James

James, after one of his earliest, post–weight loss shopping trips, offered these thoughts:

Going to a department store made me think of a shopping trip when I was 20 years old and 250 lb. I'd "outgrown" all of my shirts. It took me months to admit it. I'd already started wearing my shirts unbuttoned and a T-shirt underneath. Then I found I couldn't get my arms into the sleeves. It was a Sunday morning, and it was the only time I could bring myself to go into the store because it was pretty empty. My friends were all out at the game. I was searching the larger men's section looking at flannel jackets. There were lots of obese women there, too, looking at them. We all tried to avoid eye contact in our shame. I hurriedly bought a red checked jacket and felt even more sorry for the women.

When I lost the first 50 lb, I could downsize my trousers by two sizes, but my arms still only just barely fit into the flannel jacket. It was not until I lost another 25 lb that my arms fit comfortably in the sleeves. Unfortunately, male jacket shoulders are cut very wide and I still looked like a gorilla.

One of the hardest lessons we have to learn is to avoid any shapeless and/or oversized clothes. It is unhelpful to buy things that are already oversized when our bodies are reducing. Fabrics that stretch are always a good choice. They can contour to our bodies at a variety of sizes as we go down the weight ladder. Small prints are excellent for hiding lumps and bumps. It is best to pick the smallest size that we can possibly fit into so that we can get maximum use out of the clothes now and in the future as we maintain our new weight.

It is not just the outside layer that matters. Since undergarments are the base of every outfit, a poorly fitting bra and underpants can derail even the best clothing choices. Overweight men have known the value of a good, tight belt. Belts are also important for women because they let us turn something without shape into something more flattering by redefining our waists.

Start with buying a few basic items that are not too expensive and change them regularly as a reward, such as blue jeans and a fitted blouse or shirt. Have at least two of each "basic" piece of clothing that fits: two pairs of jeans, dress pants, suits, or skirts.

Quite often, we forget that our extremities change shape too. Buying shoes can be difficult because not only do our feet change shape, but also the way we walk and distribute our weight changes. As we lose weight and engage more in physical activity, our gait and balance improve.[19] As we near our goal weight, on average we take longer steps and narrower strides.[20] Transitioning into shoes that match our new shape can challenging. Visit a shoe store where trained employees can listen to your shoe needs and help choose a pair that will best fulfil them. Ideally, the best shoes for walking are those with a low heel, large contact area, comfortable fit, and an antislip, moderately hard sole. Walking in high heels, without shoes, or in socks increases the risk of falling.[21] So searching for the right shoes can be problematic.

It is best to wait until the afternoon to shop for shoes, as our feet naturally expand through the force of gravity and use during the day. They also swell more in hot weather. No one has the same-sized left and right feet to start with, and the differences can increase as we lose weight. Just as our bodies don't lose weight in an orderly fashion, neither do our feet. It is important to have the salesperson measure both feet—and get measured every time we buy new shoes. If one foot is larger or wider than the other, we need to buy a size that fits the larger foot and leave at least a quarter- to a half-inch of space between our longest toe and the tip of the shoe. Wearing the same type of socks or stockings that we intend to wear with the shoes will ensure that you know how the shoes will feel after leaving the shop. Spend some time walking around in the shoes to see how they feel.

Long-term excess weight places a strain on the veins that return blood from our feet. Losing weight cannot reverse that problem. So there is no point thinking, as we did when we were younger, that shoes just need to be "broken in" or that they will stretch over time. We need to find shoes that fit from the start. Shoe sizes do not always equate with shoe fit. Comfort level should be our decider.[22]

Relationships and Sex

Having a totally different body can bring up uncertainties about our emotional and sexual relationships, and things can go either way. A lot depends on how we have viewed our bodies before we achieved weight disruption. Some of us who have been overweight all our lives have never learned how to be intimate in a healthy way. Rediscovering our bodies can be exciting, and losing extra weight can affect our sex life in a positive way. Many of us find that, after we lose weight, the sensual feel of our partner's touch is heightened and that we want more frequent sex, have greater sexual desire, and even better vaginal lubrication and improvements in erectile function.[23] For others, excess skin may present a problem, but cover-up lingerie is an option to deal with that.

The Long Road

Reaching our goal weight is not the end of the story. When the tasks of weight disruption no longer consume a large amount of our thinking and actions, our capacity to respond to weight-increasing threats can diminish. For example, when we are stressed, we can experience lapses in concentration, delays in response, and distortions of judgment, all of which can add up to extra pounds in weight. At these times, prevention is better than cure. Responding to small stresses and not letting them build up can turn the negative effects of stress into motivators to maintain a healthy weight.[24]

Achieving weight disruption is a major success worth sharing. Telling others about the benefits we have accrued is also a long-term benefit for us. Table 9.1 presents a list of observations that people who have maintained a healthy weight have told me they share with others.

Table 9.1   Graduation

- My heart is in better shape—both the physical and the emotional one.
- I feel like I have something to offer others because people often ask me for weight-loss advice.
- People I haven't seen for a long time don't recognize me in the street anymore, and it is always a pleasant surprise when they say something about how good I look.
- I actually like healthy food such as salads now, and I have won my family over to thinking the same way.
- Physical activity and exercise are enjoyable parts of my daily routine and not chores.
- Trying on clothes can be enjoyable.
- Sitting in normal seats and using normal seatbelts, for example in airplanes, is very satisfying.
- My rings are easier to fit on and get off my fingers.
- My boss treats me with more respect, and my salary has also improved.
- My allergies are not so bad in the spring.
- My taste buds seem to have started working again.
- My blood pressure, diabetes, and cholesterol have improved, and I need to take fewer medications—I feel good about being heathier, and it saves me money, too.
- My memory is better.
- I sweat less.

Notes

1. http://citeseerx.ist.psu.edu/viewdoc/download?doi=10.1.1.509.1593&rep=rep1&type=pdf

2. https://academic.oup.com/ajh/article/19/11/1101/177531/Long-Term-Weight-Loss-and-Blood-Pressure-Reduction

3. http://onlinelibrary.wiley.com/doi/10.1002/oby.20944/full

4. http://www.nature.com/ijo/journal/v31/n1/full/0803363a.html

5. https://www.researchgate.net/profile/Ping_Zhang9/publication/267755698_Impact_of_an_Intensive_Lifestyle_Intervention_on_Use_and_Cost_of_Medical_Services_Among_Overweight_and_Obese_Adults_With_Type_2_Diabetes_The_Action_for_Health_in_Diabetes/links/54ae9e8c0cf29661a3d39cc3.pdf

6. http://aura.abdn.ac.uk/bitstream/handle/2164/3181/Kwok_et_al_2014_Int_J_Cardiol.pdf?sequence=1&isAllowed=y

7. http://www.obesityaction.org/educational-resources/resource-articles-2/general-articles/getting-back-in-the-game-after-significant-weight-loss

8. https://authoritynutrition.com/loose-skin-after-weight-loss

9. http://beautifulmed.it/wp-content/uploads/2016/09/AESTETIC-MEDICINE-VOL.2.pdf#page=35

10. https://www.ncbi.nlm.nih.gov/pmc/articles/PMC4241550

11. http://escholarship.org/uc/item/57q9j7p2

12. https://www.ncbi.nlm.nih.gov/pmc/articles/PMC4241550

13. https://www.intechopen.com/books/body-contouring-and-sculpting/body-contour-surgery-in-massive-weight-loss-patients

14. http://parjournal.net/article/view/1882

15. http://onlinelibrary.wiley.com/doi/10.1111/obr.12481/full

16. http://www.tandfonline.com/doi/abs/10.1080/10937404.2016.1246391#aHR0cDovL3d3dy50YW5kZm9ubGluZS5jb20vZG9pL3BkZi8xMC4xMDgwLzEwOTM3NDA0LjIwMTYuMTI0NjM5MT9uZWVkQWNjZXNzPXRydWVAQEAw

17. http://www.tandfonline.com/doi/abs/10.1080/10937404.2016.1246391#aHR0cDovL3d3dy50YW5kZm9ubGluZS5jb20vZG9pL3BkZi8xMC4xMDgwLzEwOTM3NDA0LjIwMTYuMTI0NjM5MT9uZWVkQWNjZXNzPXRydWVAQEAw

18. https://www.researchgate.net/profile/Antony_Karelis/publication/304195799_Adverse_effects_of_weight_loss_Are_persistent_organic_pollutants_a_potential_culprit/links/577aa83508ae213761c9c186.pdf

19. http://www.nejm.org/doi/full/10.1056/Nejmoa1008234#t=article

20. https://www.hindawi.com/journals/jobe/2017/4193256/abs

21. https://www.researchgate.net/profile/Tine_Roman_de_Mettelinge/publication/273833943_Does_Footwear_Matter_When_Performing_Spatiotemporal_Gait_Analysis_Among_Older_Women/links/5547522c0cf234bdb21dd6e5.pdf

22. http://www.health.harvard.edu/pain/8-tips-for-buying-shoes-that-are-good-to-your-feet

23. http://onlinelibrary.wiley.com/doi/10.1038/oby.2012.104/full

24. http://epublications.marquette.edu/cgi/viewcontent.cgi?article=1016&context=psych_fac&sei-redir=1&referer=https%3A%2F%2Fscholar.google.co.uk%2Fscholar%3Fq%3D%2522Cusp%2Bcatastrophe%2Bmodels.%2522%26btnG%3D%26hl%3Den%26as_sdt%3D0%252C5#search=%22Cusp%20catastrophe%20models.%22

CHAPTER TEN

Medical and Surgical Treatments

This chapter is about the medical and surgical ways that we can use to help us control how much we eat and drink, how much we absorb, and how much we excrete. Weight management is mainly about what we put into our mouths and what we excrete. Any medical or surgical treatment is only as good as its contribution to helping us maintain a healthy balance of intake and output. Often, overweight goes hand in hand with other medical conditions such as diabetes, high blood pressure, cholesterol problems, and arthritis. It is wise to discuss these problems with our physicians because they may affect the way we can disrupt our weight.

Many drug therapies focus on curbing our appetite or reducing our craving for food. The sensations of hunger and fullness are closely linked, and feedback loops exist in our brains to make sure we don't starve. That is why losing weight becomes difficult when we reach the set point at which our bodies say we are in energy balance, especially if that "point" is set to an unhealthy weight. Medical and surgical treatments can assist in disrupting this setting but cannot work unless our eating changes too.

We cannot predict which of us will benefit and by how much. We have to be prepared for long-term disruption.

Medications and types of surgery for obesity have come into and out of fashion as our research and knowledge have increased. Overall, the range of weight loss we can achieve from medications is between 2 and 10 kg

(4.4–22 lb), although some people can lose much more. Medications approved for long-term obesity treatment, when used with lifestyle changes such as diet and exercise, can lead to greater weight loss than just one strategy alone.[1] Unfortunately, we can't predict how drugs will work on individuals or how much weight we might lose. That is why we have to be prepared to keep on disrupting our treatments and changing them if they don't work or when they work only accompanied by unhealthy side effects.

Also, not everyone benefits from drug therapy, and none of these medications have any effect after we stop taking them. For those of us who do shed weight, most of the weight loss occurs within the first six months of

It is best to consult with an expert with regard to any drug.

therapy. If we don't lose 2 kg (4.4 lb) in the first four weeks after starting the medication, it is not working, and it is time to change it and/or alter our other activities, such as diet. In the long term, when obesity drugs work, they can increase weight loss by 3–9% more than if we don't use them. For a 70-kg (155-lb) person, that can mean a loss of over 6 kg (14 lb).[2]

The U.S. Food and Drug Administration (FDA) is the best source of information about what treatments really work. They assess all clinical trials against strict criteria, and all approved drugs must meet these criteria through clinical trials before they are approved for weight management. The FDA also requires a series of specifications to be met before they approve a drug or procedure, such as that all participants in the trials must have either a BMI≥30 (or≥27 if they have two other major health problems associated with obesity) and that over 3,000 people must be taking the drug on trial.[3]

Unfortunately, most of the evidence we have, however, is from very carefully constructed research trials and is not always applicable in the real world. There are many obstacles along the way when trying to understand the latest evidence. First, the FDA requires that the drug must result in a weight loss of over 5% more than a group not taking the drug; so very few trials compare one treatment with another. This makes it difficult to know which treatment is best. Most of us have tried several strategies before and would like to know whether and why the new drugs are better than older ones.

The FDA stipulates that, for a drug to be approved, the drug trials have to last at least one year, but we really don't know how long a trial should run to be sure that the results translate into long-term changes to weight. Most trials are very costly, so they do not continue beyond a year or two. Obesity is a lifelong problem for most of us, and we all know it is a struggle to keep the weight off over years, so the short-run results aren't helpful to us. Also, long-term side effects are not determined in these relatively short studies.

Because new drugs and clinical trials are expensive to run, the trials very tightly select people who can enter them. For example, the FDA stipulates that people enrolled in trials must have failed other weight-loss treatments, including diet and lifestyle modification.[4] In most trials, people are able to enter them only after they have tried to lose weight for six months. Most trials use 5% weight loss as a measure of success, but that metric is not helpful to those of us who have tried to lose weight several times in the past. Losing 5% of our body weight in a short time is not impossible, but maintaining that loss and losing more is the real problem. Our bodies are clever—they remember what we have tried and can work against old strategies.

Drugs can assist us to lose weight in two ways. First, drugs can control our appetite and make us feel full. They can help us regulate how often we eat, how much we eat, and how long we take to eat. They work on the part of our brain (the hypothalamus) that controls how hungry and how full we feel. The hypothalamus is the command center. It controls signals into and out from the body—mainly from our fat cells and stomach—and other parts of the brain translate those signals into appetite sensations. This a growing area of drug research. Second, they regulate how much we absorb and/or increase how much we put out, such as drugs that reduce the absorption of fat as it passes through our stomach and intestines (e.g. lipase inhibitors). Other drugs, mainly used in people with diabetes, decrease how much carbohydrate and sugars are taken in by increasing their excretion through the kidneys.[5]

FDA-Approved Strategies

Five pharmaceutical strategies are currently approved by the FDA for the treatment of obesity: orlistat, lorcaserin, liraglutide, phentermine/topiramate, and bupropion/naltrexone. Orlistat, lorcaserin, naltrexone/bupropion, phentermine/topiramate, and liraglutide all achieve at least 5% weight loss at 52 weeks. Phentermine-topiramate and liraglutide are most likely to achieve this weight loss. The most effective combination treatment seems to be the combined administration of phentermine/topiramate, followed by lorcaserin and bupropion/naltrexone.[6]

Unfortunately, not all people stay on the drugs long enough to achieve reductions. All the drugs have high dropout rates—at least one in three people.[7]

Orlistat (Xenical®, Alli®)

Orlistat works by preventing the hormone lipase from absorbing the fat we eat. It works both in the stomach and in the intestines. The extent to which orlistat blocks fat absorption is proportional to the amount of fat we eat. In most people, orlistat blocks up to 30 g fat daily when it is given as one tablet (120 mg) before meals. It is recommended for people with a BMI≥30 or with a BMI≥27 for those with other health problems like diabetes and high blood pressure. Orlistat works in two connected ways: one physical and one behavioral. Physically, it prevents us from absorbing too much fat by reducing fat absorption and causing intolerable side effects if we eat too much of it, for example more than 30 g per day. The side effects include oily spotting from the bowels, farts with a discharge, urgency to pass stools, and oily stools that don't flush away very easily. Behaviorally, when the drug works, these side effects cause us to recognize high-fat foods and modify our behavior with respect to eating fat. Side effects and cost are the main reasons people stop taking this drug. The side effects decrease over time, and by adding psyllium, which bulks up our stools, the leakage can be decreased. However, the smelly gas remains.

Orlistat, by decreasing how much fat we absorb, also decreases the amounts of vitamins A, D, E, and K that are linked to the fat to be absorbed by the body. These vitamins must be supplemented. Of the many studies looking at orlistat, perhaps the most favorable study found that, at 12 months, people on Orlistat had lost around 11 kg (24.2 lb) and, by four years, had a total reduction from the original weight of about 7 kg (15.4 lb).[8] That is roughly the same as any single nondrug weight-reduction strategy.

Lorcaserin (Belviq)

Lorcaserin works in the brain to increase our feelings of fullness so that we eat less food. It is taken twice daily in 10-mg tablets. Lorcaserin, in addition to some nutritional and exercise counseling, decreases body weight by approximately 3.2 kg (7.5 lb) (≈3.2% of initial body weight) more than people not taking it. Over two years of the clinical trial, people taking lorcaserin lost 5.6 kg (12.3 lb). Blood pressure, total cholesterol, bad cholesterol, and triglycerides also decreased. That is roughly the same as any single weight-reduction strategy. The main side effects of lorcaserin are headache, nausea, fatigue, dizziness, and back pain. There are also reports of more serious side effects, including cancer and heart valve disease.

Liraglutide (Victoza)

Liraglutide was first developed to control to type 2 diabetes. It is an injection that is used with a diet and exercise program to control blood sugar levels in adults with type 2 diabetes when other medications do not control glucose levels well enough. Then liraglutide was found to work on specific brain areas that control body weight, including the hypothalamus, even in obese people who did not have diabetes.[9] Over a year, users can expect to lose up to 6.4 kg (14 lb), and as many as 50% will lose 5% of their body weight.[10] That is roughly the same as any single weight-reduction strategy. The most common side effects are nausea, low blood sugar, diarrhea, constipation, vomiting, headache, dyspepsia, fatigue, dizziness, and abdominal pain. Severe side effects are very rare but include pancreatitis, gallbladder disease, heart rate increase, hypersensitivity reactions, and suicidal behavior. In mice and rats, liraglutide was shown to increase the risk of thyroid cancer, but this has not occurred in humans.

Phentermine/Topiramate (Qnexa, Qsiva)

Combination drugs are effective when the right ones are used because they work on different body systems and have the potential to minimize our body's counterattacks against any obesity medication. Combination therapy also means that lower doses of each medication can be prescribed, and so the side effects of each individual drug can be minimized.

Phentermine is a member of the amphetamine family and has been used in the short-term treatment of obesity for decades. It was part of a weight-loss drug combination with fenfluramine, commonly called Phen-Fen. The combination was taken off the market because fenfluramine had serious side effects on the heart and lungs.

Topiramate was developed to treat epilepsy. It was not successful at the usual doses because of serious side effects. The most serious one was that it had an association with the women taking it giving birth to children born with cleft palates. It is, however, useful in combination and smaller doses.

The phentermine and topiramate combination is the first combination of drugs for obesity to enter the market since Phen-Fen was removed. It is effective in those people who can tolerate the maximum dose of both drugs. In one year, the weight loss was 10 kg (22 lb), but only just over half the participants completed the trial. Those who did completed their second year of treatment and achieved a weight loss of 10% of their body weight. The main reasons for dropping out were blurry vision, headache, irritability, dizziness, abnormal sensation, sleeplessness, depression, and anxiety.[11]

Several groups of people should not use this combination, including women considering pregnancy or of reproductive age. The combination is also known to increase the pulse, so it is not recommended for people with unstable heart disease.

Naltrexone/Bupropion (Mysimba Contrave)

Contrave is a combination of naltrexone, which is used in the treatment of opioid addiction and alcoholism, and bupropion, which is used in the treatment of depression and smoking cessation. Naltrexone alone does not cause not weight reduction, but, with bupropion, the combination results in some weight loss. The mechanism of how they work together is not known. However, when given together, they reduce appetite and also improve the depression that can be associated with obesity. The most common side effects of bupropion are dry mouth, nausea, headache, agitation, and sleeplessness. In rare cases, it can cause serious seizures.

Other Strategies

Sibutramine

Sibutramine is a stimulant that was widely used to suppress appetite after approval by the FDA in 1997. A large study showed an increased risk of heart attack or stroke, and the FDA removed it from the market in 2010. However, sibutramine is still found illegally in some plant-based "natural" products used to manage obesity.[12]

Fenproporex (Feporex)

Fenoproporex is very similar to amphetamines. It works to block appetite by stimulating one of the hormones that make us ready to fight or run away—norepinephrine. The amount of weight loss achieved is not very large when compared with other drugs, less than 2 kg (4.4 lb) in two months and less than 5 kg (11 lb) in six months and up to one year of treatment. The most common side effects are irritability and insomnia. However, due to its serious side effects on circulation and the potential for addiction, it is not recommended by the FDA.[13] Unfortunately, fenoproporex is also found illegally in some plant-based "natural" products used to manage obesity.

Amfepramone (Anorex, Dobesin, Regenon)

Amfepramone (diethylpropion) is available in Europe for the short-term (six weeks to three months) treatment of obesity. Due to its serious side effects on the circulation and the potential for addiction, it is not recommended by the FDA. Unfortunately, amfepramone is also found illegally in some plant based "natural" products used to manage obesity.

New Drugs on the Horizon

Exenatide (Byetta, Bydureon)

Exenatide is in a class of medications called "incretin mimetics" and is largely used as an injection for diabetics. It works by stimulating the pancreas to secrete insulin. It is not yet available to treat obesity—except in clinical trials.[14] How it works in obesity is not fully understood, but it is thought to do one of three things: either slow down stomach emptying and cause a decrease in appetite; change the levels of hormones in the stomach that control appetite; or cause nausea, resulting in decreased food intake. It can result in about 5 kg (11 lb) weight loss and help to reduce daily caloric intake by 449 kcal. Other advantages of exenatide are that it works immediately and doesn't have the serious side effects common with other drugs. It can also be used long term in diabetic patients.[15] The main side effects are common: nausea and diarrhea.[16] It is available only as an injection.

No one pharmacological strategy for weight loss is effective in the long term. We have talked before about the body getting used to weight management activities and the need for disrupting the activities and changing them regularly until a lifelong pattern is achieved. That can take up to 10 years. Dependence on one type of treatment is almost always destined to fail. In the worst circumstance, it fails either by the body rejecting it or the treatment being stopped. Edie's story is an example.

Edie

Edie is now 55. She has struggled with her weight since she had her first child in her mid-thirties. She gained weight slowly but steadily, about 10 pounds a year. During her third pregnancy, she developed diabetes. For years, she tried a variety of weight-loss programs, usually losing about 10 pounds in a few weeks. She would stay in the program but always plateaued, and this made her stop. Someone told her of a new drug trial approved by FDA, and she came to me to help her get into the trial. Edie was very responsive to the medication and lost 40 pounds, almost 20% of her weight, in the first year of the trial. Unfortunately, after five years, the trial ended, and Edie no longer could get the treatment for free through the trial. Over the following year, she regained most of the weight she had lost. At her last visit to me, she said she was hopeful that the drug will come on the market soon at a reasonable price; until then, she asked me to see if I could find a supply for her—something that wasn't possible.

We discussed other methods to disrupt her weight. Together, we made a list of everything she had tried and mapped out a plan for the next decade—including the possibility that the drug might come onto the market during that time and become one of her strategies.

Like Edie, weight loss is very important for those of us who have type 2 diabetes, which is often accompanied with overweight or obesity. It is not just injections for diabetes that can help weight loss; there are now tablets for diabetes that also can assist weight loss. They are called "SLGT2 inhibitors" and include dapagliflozin (Forxiga), canagliflozin (Invokana), and empagliflozin (Jardiance). The initial weight loss is about 1–2 kg (2–4 lb), probably through the water loss that accompanies the increased amount of sugar (glucose) excreted in the urine. This weight loss continues to increase up to 2–4kg (4–9 lb) and has been shown to be maintained for up to four years—but only in clinical trials and with close supervision. The major side effects of these drugs are that they slightly increase the risk of urinary tract and genital infections.

Which Drug Is Best?

There is no perfect weight-loss medication. All available products result in short-term loss, but the loss is rarely maintained and certainly not without a diet. The important thing to remember is that our bodies get used to whatever we try. We have to keep on disrupting our strategies for maximal effect.

If we are depressed or have problems feeling full or craving certain foods, a medication that acts in our brain might be better.

If the problem is mainly in our stomach, such as too fast stomach emptying, drugs that slow down the food transit in your stomach and increase your sense of fullness, such as liraglutide, are best. Or, if the problem is that our stomachs have grown too big, drugs that make our stomach feel smaller such as bupropion/naltrexone are best.

If we are depressed or have problems feeling full or craving certain foods, medications that act in our brains, such as lorcaserin or bupropion/naltrexone, might be better. Other medications that work to reduce appetite but by a different mechanism can also work, such as phentermine/topiramate.

If we want to focus on excretion, then products that increase the fat output of our stools are best, such as orlistat.

Be Aware of Other Drugs That Unintentionally Cause Changes in Weight

Some drugs used to control other conditions can affect our weight. Commonly used drugs that cause weight gain and weight loss are listed in Tables 10.1 and 10.2.[17]

Dietary Supplements: Effects and Risks

The antiobesity mechanisms of most of medicinal plants are not clear, and often neither are their benefits or their safety. Most of the plants used in weight reduction have some antioxidant activity. *Nigella sativa, Camellia*

Table 10.1   Drugs That Can Cause Weight Gain

Drug	Condition	Amount of gain (kg)
mirtazapine	Depression	1.5
amitriptyline	Depression	1.8
nateglinide	Diabetes	0.3
sitagliptin	Diabetes	0.6
gliclazide	Diabetes	1.8
glimepiride	Diabetes	2.1
glipizide	Diabetes	2.2
glyburide	Diabetes	2.6
pioglitazone	Diabetes	2.6
tolbutamide	Diabetes	2.8
gabapentin	Pain	2.2
risperidone	Schizophrenia	0.8
quetiapine	Schizophrenia	1.1
olanzapine	Schizophrenia	2.4

Table 10.2 Drugs That Can Cause Weight Loss

Drug	Condition	Amount of loss (kg)
fluoxetine	Depression	1.3
acarbose	Diabetes	0.4
miglitol	Diabetes	0.7
metformin	Diabetes	1.1
pramlintide	Diabetes	2.3
zonisamide	Epilepsy	7.7

sinensis, green tea, and black Chinese tea were found to have acceptable antiobesity effects.[18] The effects are usually quite small and less than most diets. However, these may ultimately prove useful when we are plateauing as a temporary disruption before we start a new strategy. Unfortunately, there is little information about the side effects of these plants, and their safety still needs to be researched.[19]

Glucomannan (All Evo, Kilo Trim, XLS Medical Appetite Reducer)

Glucomannan, or konjac mannan, is dietary fiber available without prescription that increases our feelings of fullness. It forms a gel-like mass in the stomach. To achieve weight loss, at least 1 g of glucomannan should be taken three times a day with one or two glasses of water before meals. There are many unanswered questions about glucomannan. The marketed products do not display the amount of active product on the labels, and some of the components may be substances banned as dietary supplements because they are not regulated by the FDA. No studies of glucomannan have lasted longer than three months, and a recent review didn't find that glucomannan added any additional weight loss to a diet.

Cactus Fig Extract (Litramine, XLS Medical Fat Binder)

This fiber complex is made from the dry leaves of the fig cactus *Opuntia ficus-indica*. It seems that this complex gets covered with a gel in the stomach. The gel–fiber complex attracts some fat and is excreted undigested. This gel package forms a firm structure in the stomach, which is supposed to add to our feelings of fullness. After 12 weeks, people taking this complex lost at least 3% of their body weight, but there is no data on whether this was maintained.

White Bean Extract (*Phaseolus vulgaris* (XLS-Medical Carb Blocker))

A number of drugs and naturally occurring foods such as beans contain a substance, an alpha-amylase inhibitor, that reduces the energy content of food, as well as the absorption by the gut of carbohydrates. Bean extracts have been developed to increase the potency of the effect. The extract from the white bean (*Phaseolus vulgaris*) is one of them. After a 12-week trial, the weight loss was 2 kg (4 lb).[20]

Garcinia cambogia

Garcinia cambogia is a plant that grows in Southeast Asia, and its fruit has been trialed in a few studies to induce weight loss. Results of a clinical trial showed that a daily intake of 2.4 g of *Garcinia* standardized extract, with a 1,200-kcal diet taken for three months, resulted in 1.3 kg (<3 lb) weight loss—less than is achieved by any one dietary or physical activity strategy.[21]

The Synthetic Cannabis Family: Rimonabant, Taranabant

These drugs have been developed to mimic how cannabis is handled by our system, which plays a significant role in the control of our appetite as well as how we use glucose. Unfortunately, the first of these drugs, rimonabant, was associated with psychiatric side effects, including anxiety, depression, and suicidal thoughts, so it was removed from the market in 2008. The others were withdrawn from clinical trials.[22]

Herbal Medical Products: Fact or Fiction?

There is an increasing interest in herbal medical products, perhaps because the results with conventional medicines are not very promising and seem to disappear after a year or two. These products are supposed to contain exclusively herbal drugs as ingredients, such as parts of plants. It is difficult to evaluate these herbal treatments for obesity as many of them contain synthetic prescription drugs. There have been many reports of adulterated herbal supplements that were claimed to be "all natural."[23]

Many "natural" products and techniques have been proposed to induce weight loss without any evidence in humans. Table 10.3 lists a sample of such products and techniques.[24]

Beyond medications, surgical interventions can help to disrupt our weight. For example, weight-loss (bariatric) surgery is growing in importance in weight management—especially for very obese people who haven't

Table 10.3   "Natural" Weight-Loss Products and Techniques

Acupunture (of the ear)

Black wattle (*Acacia mollissima*)

Blueberry (*Vaccinium ashei*) and mulberry (*Morus australis*)

Chili pepper (*Capsicum annuum*)

Coffee (*Coffea arabica*)

Coptis Root (*Rhizoma coptidis*)

Ginger (*Zingiber officinale*)

Grapes and red wine (resveratrol)*

Green tea (*Camellia sinensis*)

Green tea (catechins especially epigallocatechin gallate)*

Lotus leaf with taurine (*Nelumbo nucifera*)

Phytosterols*

Salvia officinalis L leaves*

Shiikuwasa (*Citrus depressa*)

Soybean (*Glycine max*)

Turmeric (*Curcuma longa*)

White mulberry (*Morus alba*)

*Only theoretical evidence is available for these substances (http://www.mdpi.com/1420-3049/21/10/1404/htm).

managed to lose weight through other methods. Bariatric surgery can result in sustainable weight loss for more than five years in most patients.[25] Also, liposuction, or the removal of fat from particular regions of the body, can also be a useful technique.

Disrupting weight using medications or surgery will always involve working with physicians. When we are considering something medical or surgical, we need to be sure that our clinicians can focus beyond our acute medical problems or the consequences of overweight, such as heart disease, to a more long-term view of how to assist us to disrupt our weight. Our relationships with our physicians evolve over time and change with the ebb and flow of illness issues and familiarity.[26] We need to negotiate with our doctors in order for them to understand the fluctuating biorhythms of caring for us. Sometimes that means helping them shift from the comfort of dealing with our acute illnesses to the long-term, more difficult problem of weight disruption. Many doctors focus on disease and immediate problems but have less time to engage with us about that other complex problem, weight management—especially when weight disruption is a lifelong problem that must always be attended to and that is never "cured." A team approach to weight disruption can help.

Interventional Treatments

Surgical methods used to treat obesity are commonly referred to as "bariatric surgery." Bariatric surgery has proven to be a treatment of choice for morbid (extreme) obesity, and it is recommended for people with a BMI above 40 kg/m^2 or higher than 35 kg/m^2 when associated with other life-threatening illnesses such as diabetes.[27] The selected procedure should be relatively safe, for example with a mortality rate less than 1%. It also should reduce body weight by 50%, sustain the weight loss for at least five years, and benefit more than 75% of the people who undergo the procedure.

Bariatric operations have traditionally been divided into three groups: procedures that produce weight loss solely by limiting intake, such as gastric banding; operations that induce weight loss totally by interference with digestion and absorption, such as intestinal bypass; and procedures that both limit intake and produce malabsorption, such as gastric bypass.[28] They are more successful than diet alone in the medium term but come with a number of increased risks.

Some surgeons believe that the newer techniques done through laparoscopy are much safer than the open surgical approaches. All the procedures bring remarkable results in the short term. Weight loss within 1.5 years is between 49% and 81%. A very small group of patients have been followed up for over 10 years and showed promising results of up to 50% sustained weight loss.[29] However, the ones who weren't successful may have not come back for follow-ups. The jury is still out whether the risks outweigh the benefits.

Space-Occupying Devices: Balloons

Space-occupying devices, such as gastric balloons, are supposed to limit the size of our stomachs and make less space available to accommodate food. The idea is to help us feel full with lower amounts of food. Intragastric balloons (IGBs) have been used in the treatment of obesity for the last 20 years. These balloons are placed in the stomach through a gastroscope, that is, down a tube through the mouth, and then they are filled. The filling differs among devices but can include saltwater, dyed solution (so that leakages can be detected easily), or gas.

The original balloons were made from latex, which was not resistant to the strong acids in our stomachs, and they deflated quickly. These days they are made from acid-resistant silicone. They are usually filled with up to three glasses of saltwater and methylene blue solution. The methylene blue is added in case the balloon bursts; the dye is then excreted through the kidneys and turns the urine green. Balloons should be removed after a maximum of six months; beyond this time the risk of their spontaneously bursting is high. The procedure for balloon removal is also performed under sedation using an endoscope. The most common complications include nausea and vomiting, which can persist for up to a week in two-thirds of patients. Other adverse events include stomach ulcers and (very rarely) perforation of the stomach wall.

The balloons are taken out once the goal weight is achieved. The change in weight can be great: about 15 kg (33 lb). And the change in BMI is also quite large: up to 6. Unfortunately, only one in four maintains the weight loss for up to 30 months after the procedure. So balloon treatment, in addition to lifestyle modification, is an effective short-term procedure for weight loss. It is not surprising that there is not enough evidence confirming its long-term value because if it works for only 30 months, it can be only one temporary part of a long-term disruptive process.[30]

Adjustable Gastric Banding

An adjustable gastric band is placed through a gastroscope around the entry to the stomach in order to constrict its size. The band is connected to the outside of our body via a tube, which sits just under the skin and is called a "subcutaneous port." The size of the entry to the stomach is controlled by filling or emptying the balloon through this subcutaneous port. The aim is to reduce the amount and type of food we can eat. A well situated band will allow us to eat only about 50 g (2 oz) at a time.

Rapid weight loss is possible during the first 12 months, and after that up to 70% of the weight that is lost is often regained. For most people, the 30% weight loss is maintained for five years or longer.[31] The procedure takes less than an hour and can be done in an outpatient setting. Because the stomach is the site of absorption of some important minerals, banding can result in deficiencies in these important nutrients: iron, calcium/vitamin D, vitamin B12, copper, and thiamine. Most people will need to take some supplementation.[32]

Dolly

Recall the case of Dolly in Chapter 6. Dolly and I had spoken on the phone and skyped for a while before we met in person and I saw that she was obese—and embarrassed about it. She had even missed out on several jobs at the interview because of her size. Free of cardiovascular and orthopedic problems and not diabetic, she was the "healthy obese person."

Years later, while working together in her office, she left for the café and came back with a supersized lunch. After discussing my belief in a disruptive program, she began an exercise program, which led to health complications.

With exercise ruled out, Dolly's problem with portion size needed to be dealt with first. She had a gastric band inserted, which helped her lose 10% body weight and retrained her intake with respect to appropriate portion size. Then the band became dislodged.

Gastric bands have a number of potential problems. Bands can slip down from the neck of the stomach to the main body of the stomach and block off too much, causing swallowing problems, vomiting, and/or pain. Slipping occurs in about 5% of people who have bands inserted. If the bands slip, they need to be surgically removed. Also, bands can leak and become ineffective. The tubing can cause problems, such as the band eroding into the wall of the stomach. These difficulties occur in as many as one in every three people who have bands inserted. In the longer term, banding can cause stomach ulceration, hernias, and gallstones.

Banding can be a start in the surgical disruptive process, but it is not a long-term answer. Often bands stop working because we stop working on the other factors that keep us obese. For example, if we continue to eat large portion sizes, the part of the stomach that is higher than the band can expand and become a new absorptive place.[33]

Dolly had to have her band removed and discussed the options for more surgery with me. We agreed it was either a gastric sleeve or a gastric bypass. There are fewer complications with sleeve surgery compared with bypass. However, in the long term, there are no differences in the number of serious problems, such as reoperation, readmission to hospital, or death. Whatever procedure is done, the skill of the surgeon is very important. Surgeons in the top 25% of skill ratings have shorter operating times and fewer overall complications (5.2% versus 14.5%); lower rates of reoperation, 30-day readmission, and emergency department presentations; and fewer postoperative deaths.[34] Dolly decided to have a gastric sleeve operation at the same time the band was removed.

Gastric Sleeve

In this procedure, the stomach is reduced in size by stapling or sewing over the left part of it, so that a "sleeve" of stomach is created. Approximately

80% of the stomach is moved, creating a tube-like stomach, and that is why it is called a "sleeve." Over the past 10 years, this procedure has increased in popularity and now represents 5% of all bariatric surgery.[35] This technique works in a couple of ways to result in major weight loss. It reduces our stomach capacity and so increases a sense of fullness when we eat.

Leaking around the stitches and decreased absorption of micronutrients are the main side effects in the short term.[36] In the longer term, reflux and weight regain are the most frequent complications. Thirty percent of gastric sleeve operations require additional surgery.[37]

Roux-en-Y Gastric Bypass

This is the oldest type of surgical intervention for obesity. It was originally used for relieving blockages in the stomach and duodenum. The procedure reroutes the intestines to bypass most of the stomach and some of the small intestine. The resulting stomach is about the size of an egg and holds about 20 mL (2 T) of fluid. It requires major surgery that takes about 2 hours and is now used only when many other methods fail. The main side effects are the reduced absorption of micronutrients: calcium, iron, and vitamin B12.

A less destructive version of this technique has been developed. It is called a duodenal-jejunal bypass liner (DJBL). It is a lining that is put in place without surgery. Like the Roux-en-Y procedure, it excludes the parts of the small intestine that do most of the absorption. It is a complicated device to implant, and failure rates are as high as 20%. The main side effects are minor and include nausea and pain. However, the device can move and cause major internal problems; when that happens, it needs to be extracted.

All bypass procedures can result in side effects that are part of the process of restricting food intake. Dumping syndrome is an example, whose early symptoms (within 30 minutes after eating) occur when food and fluid pass into the small intestine too fast. The symptoms include nausea, vomiting, stomach pain or cramping, diarrhea, feelings of fullness or bloating, or increased heart rate. Later on, generally 1–3 hours after eating, decreased glucose absorption can result in flushing or sweating, an intense need to lie down, feeling weak or dizzy, feeling nervous or shaky, or a drop in blood pressure.[38]

Who Should Have Bariatric Surgery

Bariatric surgery is a very risky step in the disruptive pathway. It requires that we be well-informed of the risks and have an established commitment to weight loss; otherwise, it won't work even in the short term. Most surgeons will consider this type of surgery only if we have proven that we have lost weight by nonoperative means first, including self-directed dieting, nutritional counseling, and commercial and hospital-based weight-loss programs. Some surgeons even require us to complete a formal course of nonoperative obesity therapy before they agree to operate.[39] For adolescents, there are extra restrictions on this type of surgery. Even adolescents with a BMI >40 kg/m^2 or a BMI >35 kg/m^2 combined with severe comorbidities should be considered for surgical intervention only if they have (nearly) attained adult size. Roux-en-Y gastric bypass (RYGB) is the most effective in adolescents, probably because it has the most research data.[40] Other adolescents who should be considered for this surgery will include those who have very serious other problems that are related to their obesity, such as diabetes, sleep apnea, or severe liver disease.[41]

Some of us shouldn't consider bariatric surgery. Chronic weight losers end up stuck in cycles of weight gain and loss.[42] It is easy to think that surgery will be our final cure. Unfortunately, the risks for certain groups outweigh the benefits; for example, bariatric surgery should not be offered to the very young and the very old, people who have medical conditions that make surgery risky (such as uncontrolled diabetes), people who have severe mental health problems, and adolescents who haven't reached their full adult growth. Pregnant and lactating women shouldn't be considered for surgery or women planning for a pregnancy within two years of the surgery because the disruptive effects may affect the pregnancy.[43] Previous abdominal surgery may also make it difficult for the surgeons but doesn't rule out discussing it as an option. (See Table 10.4.)

Experimental Techniques

A number of newer techniques are under investigation. It is early, and there is no definitive answer as to how well these techniques work or for how long.

1. *Duodenal mucosal ablation* involves destroying the lining of the first part of the small intestine, the duodenum, by high-frequency radio waves. Once this has occurred, a less absorptive lining of the small intestine replaces it.

2. Injecting *Botox* into the lining of the stomach is another experimental technique. Botox partially paralyses the muscles of the stomach, causing decreased stomach contractions and therefore a heightened sense of fullness. Multiple injections are required.

3. *Gastric stimulation* involves stimulating the stomach to contract by passing an electric current through it. This can also have an effect on how full we feel after eating.

4. *Gastric artery embolization* targets the production of hormones in the stomach, such as ghrelin, that make us feel hungry. This is achieved by using microbeads to block specific arteries that carry blood to the stomach. The procedure is done under X-ray guidance without any invasive surgery. The average weight loss after six months is over 8% of body weight.[44]

5. In *intermittent vagal blockade*, rather than blocking the arteries, the nerves to the stomach can instead be intermittently blocked. The idea behind an intermittent blockade is that it avoids the body getting used to the nerves being permanently blocked.

6. *Incisionless magnetic compression anastomoses* uses self-assembling magnets to connect to various parts of the small bowel. Once one of the magnets is in place, another one is attached to an area on the corresponding other side of the small bowel. The magnets attract and try to attach to each other, causing the tissues around the magnets to die and the small bowel to remodel itself to make another route to transport food.

7. *Aspiration therapy* is a relatively new technique that diverts food out of the stomach and out of the body a short time after eating. It is a drastic short-term measure for those people who cannot stop putting food in their mouths. A tube is placed in the stomach and leads outside the body. It flushes about 30% of an eaten meal out of the stomach. The technique is very difficult for people to continue with for long periods. At six months, people who were able to complete the program were able to lose 15 kg (33 lb). It has a major effect on important body mineral absorption and is not recommended long term.

Table 10.4   Bariatric Surgery Quick Checklist

Are you morbidly obese?

Have you tried a variety of other methods? For how long?

Do you have other life-threatening problems? Diabetes?

Have you checked on the facility that will perform the procedure?

> Is it a recognized center performing at least 150 bariatric surgeries a year with a multidisciplinary team, for example a dietician, counselor, surgeon?
>
> Does your surgeon perform at least 50 operations a year?
>
> Is there long-term follow-up?

Can you afford it?

> On average, bariatric surgery costs between $15,000 and $25,000 or more, depending on what type of surgery you have and whether there are follow-up problems. Some insurers require you to show that you meet requirements first; for example, you were unable to lose weight by completing a nonsurgical weight-loss program.[*]

[*]https://www.niddk.nih.gov/health-information/health-topics/weight-control/bariatric
-surgery/Pages/definition-facts.aspx

Factoring in the Medical Problems Associated with Obesity

Many medical problems are associated with obesity. Most of the medical conditions that accompany obesity are long-term problems—just like obesity. However, dealing with them all at once is not necessary.[45] But, for safety, your doctor must be aware of any that affect you—as well as the medications you take for them—before embarking on any medical, herbal, or surgical venture to assist weight loss.

Some of these medical problems are directly related to excess weight, such as diabetes, while others occur but may not be directly related to obesity, such as arthritis. Even more common are conditions that interact with obesity, such as depression, asthma, and diabetes. Each one of these conditions can cause the other. It is important that we make sure all of these problems and potential problems are addressed with a physician before any diets, drugs, substances, or surgeries are undertaken.

Asthma

Asthma and obesity are interlinked. Although most asthma is caused by allergies, we now know that asthma accompanying obesity is not always caused by allergies.[46] Both asthma and obesity can be a cause of the other and also make each other worse. Fat around the abdomen may make breathing difficult, and the steroid inhalers used in the treatment of asthma are less effective in obese and overweight people.[47]

Arthritis[48]

Arthritis and obesity are also interlinked. Each 1-kg (2-lb) increase in weight causes an increased risk of osteoarthritis of the knees and wrists. Not only is obesity associated with an increased risk of osteoarthritis, but weight loss is associated with a decreased risk of osteoarthritis. Decreasing our BMI by 2 kg/m² can decrease our risk of osteoarthritis by 50%. Osteoarthritis that is associated with obesity occurs in both weight-bearing and non-weight-bearing joints. This suggests that obesity causes problems by increasing wear and tear not only on weight-bearing joints but also in cartilage and bone.

Cancer[49]

Overweight and inactivity account for up to a third of all cancers of the breast, colon, endometrium, kidney, and esophagus. Obesity also almost doubles our likelihood of dying from cancer and can also affect treatment.

Doses of chemotherapy are commonly reduced because of the effect of obesity on the liver, where most chemotherapy is broken down. Fortunately, effective screening programs are available to all for breast, cervical, prostate, and colon cancers. Screening mammography, however, may have to be supplemented with ultrasound for large breasts.

Diabetes

Among the complications of obesity, the most common and serious is type 2 diabetes.[50] Diabetes is a problem related to insufficient insulin, which is our main controller of energy usage and storage. When we eat protein or carbohydrate, insulin is released from the pancreas and in turn increases our absorption of both of these foods and also arranges for the storage of the energy in them for later use. Weight gain precedes the development of diabetes. The overnutrition that accompanies obesity can stress our bodies to such a degree that we become resistant to the effects of insulin. We produce more and more insulin, but it has less and less effect. Eventually, the pancreas burns out and stops producing insulin altogether. That is how type 2 diabetes occurs.

Diseases of the Heart and Circulation[51]

We know that heart disease is linked to overweight and obesity. Women who gain 5–9.9 kg (11–22 lb) are two times more likely to get high blood pressure, and men who gain 25 kg (55 lb) are five times more likely. While we know that heart disease is linked to overweight and obesity, moderate weight loss does improve life expectancy when measured at 10 years.[52] For each unit change in BMI, our risk of a heart attack increases by 10%. Eleven percent of the cases of heart failure in men and 14% in women are caused by obesity.

Gynecological and Obstetric Problems

Obesity is the cause of infertility in 6% of cases, much of it as a result of polycystic ovary syndrome (PCOS). Women with PCOS find their problems improve when they lose weight. During pregnancy, obesity is associated with an increased risk of associated diabetes (gestational diabetes) and associated high blood pressure (pre-eclampsia). Childbirth is also more problematic, with delivery complications such as enlarged heads (macrosomia) and shoulder presentations, leading to higher rates of caesarean sections.

Gum Disease

Periodontal (gum) disease is more severe and may be more common if we are overweight and have been smokers and/or have diabetes. Unfortunately, no one treatment has shown long-term promise in treating gum disease. It is best to discuss this possibility with your dentist.[53]

Liver and Gallbladder Diseases[54]

Men and women with a BMI greater than 45 kg/m² have a sevenfold increase in risk for gallstones. When we lose weight rapidly, we also have an increased risk of gallstones. Gallstone formation after bariatric surgery affects more than one in three people.

Nonalcoholic fatty liver disease (NAFLD) is also a condition that occurs as a direct result of obesity and overweight. It can lead to problems with cholesterol and triglycerides and even liver cancer. NAFLD improves with weight reduction, and for some people a greater than 5% weight reduction can return the liver to normal.

Low Testosterone

Men who are obese and also have diabetes have lower levels of testosterone. There is also a link between impotence and increasing infertility with abdominal obesity.

Mental Health Disorders[55]

Obesity can be linked with a variety of mood changes, with depression and anxiety being the most common.[56] We don't always know which comes first, but we do know that each can cause the other and make it worse.[57]

Eating disorders, such as binge eating disorder and night eating syndrome, have been linked with depression and obesity.

Mental disorders can sometimes be a cause for seeking more invasive approaches to obesity, such as bariatric surgery.

Obstructive Sleep Apnea (OSA)[58]

When fat is deposited around the neck, it is up to 10 times more likely that we will develop obstructive sleep apnea (OSA). Over 75% of patients with OSA are greater than 120% of their ideal body weight. Increased fat deposits in tissues surrounding our upper airways can directly block the trachea or breathing tube or cause our breathing tubes to collapse. Sleep apnea treatment, such as continuous positive airway pressure machines and oral appliances, is readily available these days. Significant weight loss improves but rarely cures severe obstructive sleep apnea.[59]

Not everyone who is obese will develop complications. Many factors come into play, such as physical activity, fat distribution, and family history. The age at which we become obese matters because there is a higher risk of developing obesity-related problems the earlier we become obese.

Medical Problems of Obese Children and Adolescents

The health problems associated with obesity in children and adolescents need special attention because they can progress more rapidly in these age groups, and permanent damage can occur. Because adolescence is a time of great disruption to our bodies and minds, it is a perfect time to intervene and make significant changes. Like adults, children with serious weight problems are more likely to suffer from the adult type of diabetes. However, in children, the deterioration is much faster. High blood pressure and high cholesterol are also problems.[60]

Because our fat cells are hormonal glands and can house our sex hormones, obesity can be associated with the excess production of these hormones in adolescents. Girls can become sexually mature earlier, and, as they become adolescents, they can develop problems with the balance of estrogen and testosterone, leading to polycystic ovaries, severe acne, and excess facial hair. Other skin problems are also common—rashes in skin folds, boils, and stretch marks.

As with adults who are overweight or obese, breathing problems such as sleep apnea and asthma are also more common. Nonalcoholic fatty liver disease, which is now the most common cause of liver disease in children, is also more common in obese children. Fortunately, early liver disease can be reversed with weight loss.

Excess weight can cause problems for muscles and bones, such as back and joint pain, and bowlegs.

Even when there is an effective intervention in childhood, some health problems persist. For example, mental health problems, including poor self-esteem, anxiety, and depression, often continue into adulthood even with adequate treatment of obesity in childhood.

Doctors are very good at focusing on these diseases, and there are specialty clinics for children and adolescents who have a combination of health problems. Unfortunately, the focus is usually on managing these serious problems, but preventive activities, such as contraceptive advice or smoking cessation, often are forgotten.

Too Many Problems: Where Do We Start?

A good way of looking at managing more than one associated problem is to focus on where we can get results that encourage us to keep on trying, disrupting, and succeeding. We need to negotiate this strategy with a physician to ensure that it works for us and is not something that we have tried and hasn't worked. Of the many different strategies, here are a few that physicians have shared.

Dr. Chris

Dr. Chris always aims for a treatment that can show immediate results, such as lower blood pressure. With blood pressure under control, she feels that her patients are less stressed and freer to focus on more challenging long-term problems. "I'd like to go after something I can 'fix' before the next face-to-face consultation. Since we have achieved something together, maybe this will help us plan a disruptive long-term strategy together."

Dr. Krish

He worries that a lot of his patients have heard it all before and have entirely lost hope of achieving any sustained weight loss. For these patients, he asks them what they would like to tackle first with him. Establishing trust and confidence at the outset is most important.

> I think some patients come into my room already with a closed mind. Their eyes tell you, they don't want to discuss their weight, just their diabetes or sore knees. I don't want to lose them even before we start. We have time to pick the right consultation. The last thing I would tell them is that are morbidly obese, because they know it. Telling them they really need to lose 25 pounds before we meet next time is what they have heard for years. They can do that, but it always comes back on. We have time to pick the right time to talk about sustaining change.

Drs. Izzy and Lola

The costs of being obese, compared to the costs of weight-reduction programs, can be a motivator. Drs. Izzy and Lola motivate their patients in this way. They tell them that if they can get their weight to a healthy range, they can save money on medications, health insurance, and more.

Weight reduction is the cheapest option in health care and one our patients can control. Some of my patients who are obese don't have arthritis and diabetes, and they are active. We have a hard time convincing them that because they are above insurance companies' tables for weight, they need to do something about it. Then we talk costs. They can't control the price of cholesterol and blood pressure medications, but they can control the price and the types of foods they buy and eat.

Notes

1. http://jamanetwork.com/journals/jama/fullarticle/1774038

2. http://jamanetwork.com/journals/jama/fullarticle/1774038?issueno=1&quiz=5

3. http://onlinelibrary.wiley.com/doi/10.1111/obr.12465/full

4. http://www.nature.com/ijo/journal/v40/n7/full/ijo201669a.html

5. http://onlinelibrary.wiley.com/doi/10.1111/obr.12465/full

6. http://www.sciencedirect.com/science/article/pii/S0165614716300220

7. http://jamanetwork.com/journals/jama/article-abstract/2528211

8. http://www.obesitymedicinejournal.com/article/S2451-8476(16)30001-X/fulltext#sec1.1

9. http://www.fda.gov/downloads/AdvisoryCommittees/CommitteesMeeting Materials/Drugs/EndocrinologicandMetabolicDrugsAdvisoryCommittee /UCM421474.pdf

10. http://onlinelibrary.wiley.com/doi/10.1111/obr.12465/full

11. https://www.researchgate.net/profile/Daniel_Riche/publication/242016743 _New_Obesity_Agents_Lorcaserin_and_PhentermineTopiramate_(JulyAugust) /links/53d6db6f0cf228d363ea8bda.pdf

12. https://www.researchgate.net/profile/Andre_Bairros/publication/44601590 _A_new_method_for_the_simultaneous_determination_of_14-benzodiazepines _and_amfepramone_as_adulterants_in_phytotherapeutic_formulations_by _voltammetry/links/5446bca10cf22b3c14e0b164.pdf

13. http://www.scielosp.org/scielo.php?pid=S0034-89102016000200503&script =sci_arttext

14. https://medlineplus.gov/druginfo/meds/a605034.html

15. https://www.ncbi.nlm.nih.gov/pmc/articles/PMC3495586

16. http://onlinelibrary.wiley.com/doi/10.1111/obr.12465/full

17. http://press.endocrine.org/doi/abs/10.1210/jc.2014-3421#sthash.B56LVcFy .dpuf

18. https://jdmdonline.biomedcentral.com/articles/10.1186/2251-6581-12-28

19. http://journals.sagepub.com/doi/pdf/10.1177/2156587215599105

20. http://curis.ku.dk/ws/files/156451186/Tonstad_et_al_Obesity_Medicine_2016_Vol_1_38_44.pdf

21. http://journals.sagepub.com/doi/pdf/10.1177/2156587215599105

22. https://link.springer.com/article/10.1007/s00228-013-1473-0

23. https://www.thieme-connect.com/products/ejournals/html/10.1055/s-0042-103495

24. https://pdfs.semanticscholar.org/d72c/c068e46a9e387ac4a623fa4134782f3a3d3e.pdf

25. https://www.nhlbi.nih.gov/files/docs/guidelines/prctgd_c.pdf

26. https://thethinker.co/2015/09/21/the-doctor-patient-relationship-is-on-the-rocks-is-it-time-for-couples-counseling

27. https://www.ncbi.nlm.nih.gov/pmc/articles/PMC4716069

28. https://www.ncbi.nlm.nih.gov/pmc/articles/PMC2729256

29. https://www.ncbi.nlm.nih.gov/pmc/articles/PMC4934447/pdf/mjiri-30-354.pdf

30. http://link.springer.com/article/10.1007/s11695-016-2307-9

31. http://circres.ahajournals.org/content/118/11/1844#sec-2

32. https://www.ncbi.nlm.nih.gov/pmc/articles/PMC4934447/pdf/mjiri-30-354.pdf

33. https://www.ncbi.nlm.nih.gov/pmc/articles/PMC4934447/pdf/mjiri-30-354.pdf

34. https://www.researchgate.net/profile/Emma_Osland/publication/295083820_Postoperative_Early_Major_and_Minor_Complications_in_Laparoscopic_Vertical_Sleeve_Gastrectomy_LVSG_Versus_Laparoscopic_Roux-en-Y_Gastric_Bypass_LRYGB_Procedures_A_Meta-Analysis_and_Systematic_Review/links/5848ac2f08ae61f75de35728/Postoperative-Early-Major-and-Minor-Complications-in-Laparoscopic-Vertical-Sleeve-Gastrectomy-LVSG-Versus-Laparoscopic-Roux-en-Y-Gastric-Bypass-LRYGB-Procedures-A-Meta-Analysis-and-Systematic-Review.pdf

35. http://www.sciencedirect.com/science/article/pii/S2444866416300666

36. http://www.sciencedirect.com/science/article/pii/S0016510715027418

37. http://www.sciencedirect.com/science/article/pii/S2444866416300666

38. https://www.ncbi.nlm.nih.gov/pmc/articles/PMC2939109

39. https://www.ncbi.nlm.nih.gov/pmc/articles/PMC2729256

40. http://link.springer.com/article/10.1007/s11695-015-1581-2

41. http://www.aahs.org/medstaff/wp-content/uploads/ChildhoodObesityMCP2017.pdf

42. https://thethinker.co/2017/01/09/the-obesity-epidemic-are-we-stuck-in-the-middle

43. https://www.ncbi.nlm.nih.gov/pmc/articles/PMC2939109

44. http://www.sciencedirect.com/science/article/pii/S1743919116309657

45. https://dukespace.lib.duke.edu/dspace/bitstream/handle/10161/12382/Funk%202016%20PCP%20decision%20making%20regarding%20severe%20obesity%20tx%20and%20bariatric%20surgery%20SOARD.pdf?sequence=1

46. http://www.atsjournals.org/doi/full/10.1164/rccm.201401-0178OC

47. https://academic.oup.com/qjmed/article/99/9/565/2258973/The-medical
-complications-of-obesity

48. https://academic.oup.com/qjmed/article/99/9/565/2258973/The-medical
-complications-of-obesity

49. https://academic.oup.com/qjmed/article/99/9/565/2258973/The-medical
-complications-of-obesity

50. https://www.ncbi.nlm.nih.gov/pubmed/26819198

51. https://academic.oup.com/qjmed/article/99/9/565/2258973/The-medical
-complications-of-obesity

52. http://www.ginecoweb.com/PDF/Obesidad_NEJM_2017.pdf

53. http://care.diabetesjournals.org/content/40/Supplement_1/S25

54. https://academic.oup.com/qjmed/article/99/9/565/2258973/The-medical
-complications-of-obesity

55. https://academic.oup.com/qjmed/article/99/9/565/2258973/The-medical
-complications-of-obesity

56. http://www.ginecoweb.com/PDF/Obesidad_NEJM_2017.pdf

57. http://www.nature.com/npp/journal/v42/n1/full/npp2016123a.html

58. https://academic.oup.com/qjmed/article/99/9/565/2258973/The-medical
-complications-of-obesity

59. http://www.ginecoweb.com/PDF/Obesidad_NEJM_2017.pdf

60. http://www.aahs.org/medstaff/wp-content/uploads/ChildhoodObesityMCP
2017.pdf

Appendix: Finding a Weight Control Clinician

Finding a reputable obesity clinician or service is not always an easy venture, but it is simplified by breaking it down into stages. The first step is to check whether the physician of your choice is actually educated to the recognized U.S. standard. All physicians educated in the United States must complete four years of medical school.[1] After that, U.S. medical students sit for examinations to earn their doctor of medicine (MD) degree. Doctors who attend medical school outside the United States are certified here by the Educational Commission for Foreign Medical Graduates.[2] Overseas medical degrees are not always MDs. For example, in the UK, the medical degree is a bachelor of medicine (MB) and a bachelor of surgery (BS) and can take up to six years, and an MD in the UK is equivalent to a PhD.

After medical school, physicians can take several years to gain specialty certification. A range of specialties look after people who are obese, such as family medicine, endocrinology, cardiology, obesity medicine, pediatric obesity, bariatric surgery, and plastic surgery. These physicians must pass exams and must participate in continuing education to gain and maintain their certification.[3] There are dedicated organizations that certify their ongoing learning. For example, the American Medical Association (AMA) has a Physician's Recognition Award for physicians who have completed 50 or more hours of continuing medical education annually.[4] More than 840,000 physicians are Board Certified by the AMA. Physicians can hold one or more licenses to practice medicine in the 54 U.S. licensing jurisdictions.[5]

You have a right to expect that the certifications held by your physician represent a sufficient current level of knowledge, skills, and experience to provide quality care for you. However, when you select a physician for your care or to care for someone in your family, you should be looking for more—a physician you can trust and who has the skills you need. Think of your physician as an expert who wants to be your health care partner.

Working in the field of obesity is extremely satisfying on both an intellectual and a personal level for clinicians, so most of us are motivated to help. Our patients come from all walks of life, all ages, different cultures, and varying levels of functionality. From a scientific perspective, it is also extremely interesting because lots of new information is coming out from research. If your clinician isn't motivated and reaching out to help you succeed, many others are willing do so.

> *When you select a physician, you should be looking for someone you can trust who has the skills you need.*

A couple of basic principles can assist your choice among professionals who can help. The clinician you choose has to "fit"—just like a pair of shoes. If you have a size 7 foot, not all size 7 shoes feel comfortable. You may need to do a little shopping around to find the best fit. Relationships, like shoe fit, change over time. You may find your clinician no longer has the expertise you need; for example, a family physician does not perform bariatric surgery. These changes need to be managed so that you still are getting optimal care.

Julie

Julie went to see her family doctor about losing weight. For several years after the children went to school, she had been thinking about it. Last year, her doctor told her that she had both high cholesterol and high blood pressure and that she would be on medication for life if she didn't lose weight. Julie decided it was time to take action. She wanted to lose weight quickly to be able to get into a pretty dress for her daughter's wedding and wanted her doctor to refer her to a surgeon for a gastric sleeve.

Julie's doctor explained that surgery was used only as a last resort and that she had to have a trial of strict dieting first. Julie was unhappy and decided to seek advice from another doctor. Eventually, after seeing several doctors, she was referred to a private clinic in Mexico.

Our expectations can make us impatient with clinicians. Often, we want them to provide us with an instant fix. With obesity, that is not always possible. An open and frank discussion in the beginning about long-term expectations can be helpful. Otherwise, like Julie, you can end up shopping around for a treatment that may not be appropriate from a clinician who may not have the necessary expertise.

Many organizations lay down criteria for clinical skills. For example, the Academy for Eating Disorders has a series of core skills that are essential for any clinician who wants to specialize in obesity medicine.[6] They include an understanding of obesity as a complex disease, how to assess it, and what constitutes optimal care outcomes. They recommend seeing a group of clinicians with differing skills because optimal results cannot be fully achieved by a single health professional.

The environment in which the practitioners work must also be suitable for patients with obesity. For example, appropriate parking, furniture, chairs, examination tables, and privacy when being weighed are all important considerations.

Many organizations endorse these competencies and expect their members to comply. They include:

- Academy of Nutrition and Dietetics,
- Accreditation Council for Graduate Medical Education,
- American Academy of Family Physicians,
- American Academy of Pediatrics,
- American Association of Colleges of Nursing,
- American Association of Colleges of Osteopathic Medicine,
- American Association of Colleges of Pharmacy,
- American Board of Obesity Medicine,
- American Council of Academic Physical Therapy,
- American Dental Education Association,
- American Kinesiology Association,
- American Psychological Association,
- Association for Prevention Teaching and Research,
- Association of American Medical Colleges,
- Association of Schools and Programs of Public Health,
- Centers for Medicare and Medicaid Services,
- Interprofessional Education Collaborative,
- National Organization of Nurse Practitioner Faculties,
- Physician Assistant Education Association,
- Society for Public Health Education,
- Society of Teachers of Family Medicine,
- The Obesity Society.

Choosing a clinician from any one of these groups is a good start. However, some key organizations focus specifically on obesity. Each has a specific focus, and all of them provide resources that can help you in your choices. The Obesity Society, for example, supports research on the causes, treatment, and prevention of obesity, as well as keeping the scientific community and public informed of advances in the field.[7] The Obesity Action Coalition (OAC) focuses on representing individuals affected by obesity in a number of ways, from advocating on

Capitol Hill for access to obesity treatments to publishing educational resources for the individuals affected.[8] The American Society of Metabolic and Bariatric Surgery (ASMBS) aims to improve the care and treatment of people with obesity and related diseases by advancing the science and understanding of metabolic surgery.[9] Similarly the Obesity Medicine Association (OMA), formerly the American Society of Bariatric Physicians, is the oldest medical association dedicated to the surgical treatment of obesity and associated diseases. The Academy of Nutrition and Dietetics (formerly the American Dietetic Association), the world's largest organization of food and nutrition professionals, works on improving the nation's health through advancing the profession of dietetics.

Certification of Obesity Practitioners

Obesity experts do not have to be physicians or have certification. However, some certification of skills and competency, as well as a commitment to ongoing education and training, usually means that a practitioner is actively ensuring she or he is being effective. Several bodies specifically certify obesity practitioners. The American Board of Obesity Medicine (ABOM), for example, maintains standards for the assessment and credentialing of obesity physicians.[10] Certification as an ABOM diplomate "signifies specialized knowledge in the practice of obesity medicine and distinguishes a physician as having achieved competency in obesity care." The Obesity Society regularly publishes a list of graduates of the ABOM.[11] Similarly, the Obesity Medicine Association awards fellowships to a range of clinicians, including physicians, nurse practitioners, or physician assistants who have demonstrated an ongoing commitment to the practice of obesity medicine.[12] All fellows must complete at least 75 hours of advanced training in obesity medicine. Their site contains a directory to help you search for a clinician. Also, the Certification Board for Obesity Educators credentials any qualified healthcare professional who treats obese patients.[13]

The Academy of Nutrition and Dietetics supports an interdisciplinary board-certified specialist in obesity and weight management certification. Current certification extends to nurse practitioners, exercise physiologists, dietitian nutritionists, clinical psychologists, clinical social workers, and physician assistants. Certification requires a minimum of two years of supervised practice prior to taking the exam and 2,000 hours of specialty practice experience within the past five years.

The American Council on Exercise (ACE) trains weight management specialists. The course is designed for experienced health and fitness professionals certified with ACE and other organizations, such as nurse practitioners, registered dietitians, medical assistants, community leaders, and members of the allied health team.[14]

The certification of nurse practitioners is not as clearly delineated. The American Academy of Nurse Practitioners National Certification Board provides a valid and reliable program for entry-level nurse practitioners, in order to recognize their education, knowledge, and professional expertise, as well as a process for validating an advanced practice nurse's qualifications and knowledge for practice as a nurse practitioner. The academy, however, doesn't have a particular specialty practice group on weight management. Several specialty groups, such as endocrine and cardiology, cover aspects of weight management.

Bariatric nursing, however, has a specialized training program. The Certified Bariatric Nurse (CBN) program is designed to assess the professional competence of practitioners of bariatric nursing. Bariatric nurses are certified after completing a minimum of 24 months (within the preceding four years) of nursing care of morbidly obese and bariatric surgery patients.

Also, many international organizations provide training and certification in obesity. The World Obesity Federation represents professional members of the scientific, medical, and research communities from over 50 regional and national obesity associations. The SCOPE (Specialist Certification of Obesity Professional Education) Certification is an internationally recognized standard of obesity management expertise that promotes and acknowledges excellence in obesity prevention and treatment.[15] This obesity qualification is awarded by SCOPE to healthcare practitioners who have completed the SCOPE training program. These programs are of great importance if you are considering undergoing obesity treatment outside the United States.

Julie

Julie did a lot of homework on the Internet. She found out the range of skills and training required of bariatric surgeons. She used the American Society for Metabolic and Bariatric Surgery (ASMBS) Web site to scope an appropriate set of skills, such as training in laparoscopic gastric bypass, laparoscopic adjustable gastric banding, sleeve gastrectomy, and revisional bariatric and foregut surgery.[16] In addition, ASMBS requires accredited surgeons to work in an accredited bariatric surgical center.[17]

All of the U.S. clinics that Julie contacted required her to undergo at least six months of specialized dieting before they would consider surgery. That was too long for Julie, so she decided to travel outside the United States for her surgery.

Medical tourism for obesity treatment, especially bariatric surgery, is becoming more common. There are many reasons for this migration, including lower costs, no need for medical insurance, and short or no waiting times. Americans and Canadians mainly travel to Mexico and Latin America, where treatment prices can be incredibly low, with high-quality, English-speaking clinics in exciting unusual destinations. Thailand, Singapore, and Malaysia are also very popular destinations.

Julie developed a checklist. Her first step was to identify the best-value countries for bariatric surgery. She discovered a whole series of hidden costs, such as travel and accommodation. Some places, like India, had low treatment costs but high airfares. Also, travel insurance varied from country to country. She found a

UK site called Treatment Abroad, which helped her to identify the countries with the lowest treatment prices.[18] She chose Mexico and then went about getting quotes from the actual clinics.

Reputable clinics should have Web sites that will give you all the details you need about the facilities, the services, and the consultants and surgeons on the team. The more detail they provide, the better. Cross-checking this information against other sources, such as the national health organization of the country or country-specific professional associations, is essential. Any clinic should provide you with a quote for your treatment based on your medical history. Get your quote in writing, by post or e-mail, and make sure it includes what is and is not provided.

Julie found the process very time-consuming and opted for a broker (medical agent) to get an all-inclusive quote that included arranging flights, hotels, and treatment. The broker provided customer feedback from other medical tourists, and, as well, Julie found feedback on the independent forums. These forums cited a range of pitfalls to watch out for, such as outdated equipment and techniques, poor English communication skills (especially true for South East Asians locations), prioritizing the holiday aspects rather than the technical expertise, and lack of rapid access to emergency facilities.

Medicine is not always predictable; things can go wrong with treatment abroad, which can delay your return home and result in additional health, personal, and medical costs. You should prepare for these possibilities and even consider taking along a partner or companion, if you choose this option. Follow-up back in the United States is vital, so it is important to let your home clinician know what you are going to do, so that you can plan follow-up visits upon your return.

Notes

1. https://apps.ama-assn.org/doctorfinder/html/physcred.jsp#foreign
2. https://apps.ama-assn.org/doctorfinder/html/physcred.jsp#foreign
3. https://apps.ama-assn.org/doctorfinder/html/physcred.jsp#specialty
4. https://apps.ama-assn.org/doctorfinder/html/physcred.jsp#award
5. http://www.abms.org
6. https://www.lsuhsc.edu/administration/academic/cipecp/docs/Provider-Competencies-for-the-Prevention-and-Management-of-Obesity(1).pdf
7. www.obesity.org
8. www.obesityaction.org
9. www.asmbs.org
10. http://abom.org
11. http://www.obesity.org/education/abom-certification
12. https://obesitymedicine.org/find-obesity-treatment
13. http://www.obesityeducator.org

14. https://www.acefitness.org/fitness-certifications/specialty-certifications/weight-management.aspx?gclid=CLii6NOM0dQCFeG77QodkrIPyA

15. http://www.worldobesity.org/scope/certification

16. http://asmbs.org/professional-education/cbn

17. https://www.facs.org/search/bariatric-surgery-centers

18. https://www.treatmentabroad.com

Annotated Bibliography

Sources, General Articles, and Books

Center for Nutrition Policy and Promotion. Interactive Healthy Eating Index

https://www.cnpp.usda.gov/healthyeatingindex

The Interactive Healthy Eating Index is a Web tool for consumers that allows users to enter the foods they have eaten and the physical activities they have completed in the last 24 hours. It then calculates how these foods fit into the food pyramid, how the nutrients break down, and how many calories they expended by the activity.

MedlinePlus

https://medlineplus.gov/healthstatistics.html

Provides access to information produced by the National Library of Medicine and the National Institutes of Health. There is also a database of drug and supplement information, an illustrated medical encyclopedia, a medical dictionary, links to other Web sites, and health news.

National Heart, Lung, and Blood Institute. *The Practical Guide: Identification, Evaluation, and Treatment of Overweight and Obesity.* Bethesda, MD: National Heart, Lung, and Blood Institute, 2000 (94 pp.). Sudocs Number: HE 20.3208:P 88

This is a guide intended for physicians; however, the information it contains is useful to anyone. It covers most of the general methods for assessing obesity and managing it through diet, physical activity, behavior therapy, and pharmacology. There are brief guides, such as for healthy eating out and activity diaries.

Partners in Information Access for the Public Health Workforce

https://phpartners.org/obesity.html

A collaboration of U.S. government agencies, public health organizations, and health sciences libraries to provide access to selected public health resources. It has obesity and nutrition areas, and you sign up for e-mail alerts on the latest obesity news.

Introduction

Haslam, W. D., Arya M. Sharma, and Carel W. le Roux (eds.). *Controversies in Obesity*. London: Springer-Verlag, 2014 (295 pp.).

> http://mediendo.cn/uploadfiles/kejian/20140728/0728163529_1319.pdf#page=71

> The umbrella term "obesity" does not, as it implies, equal one successful treatment and a single long-term maintenance plan. Obesity is a constellation of complex problems that grow slowly in our minds and bodies and that require a range of strategies. This book deals with a whole range of issues where there is so much uncertainty from societal issues to treatment controversies.

Chapter One

Adaptive thermogenesis in adipocytes: Is beige the new brown?

> http://genesdev.cshlp.org/content/27/3/234.full.pdf+html
> and

Turning WAT into BAT

> http://www.bioscirep.org/content/ppbioscirep/33/5/e00065.full.pdf

> Energy balance is at the center of our understanding about obesity. This means that we cannot gain or lose weight unless there is an imbalance between food intake and energy expenditure. When energy intake chronically exceeds energy expenditure, weight gain and obesity result. These articles describe the three types of fat that we have in our bodies—white, beige, and brown. It describes evidence on how we can move our fat from the toxic, energy-sparing white variety to the less toxic, energy-expending beige and further on to brown fat, which helps us stay lean.

The average caloric expenditure during an Olympic triathlon

> http://healthyeating.sfgate.com/average-caloric-expenditure-during-olympic-triathlon-12425.html

> This article compares the average calories burned in the three parts of a triathlon. It is interesting to see how much exercise is required to burn calories. The article forms the basis of the argument that exercise alone cannot induce sustained weight loss.

Chapter Two

Direct comparisons of commercial weight-loss programs on weight, waist circumference, and blood pressure: A systematic review

> https://bmcpublichealth.biomedcentral.com/articles/10.1186/s12889-016-3112-z
>
> and

Benefits of commercial weight-loss programs on blood pressure and lipids: A systematic review

> http://www.sciencedirect.com/science/article/pii/S0091743516301530
>
> Both articles are based on reviews of commercially available weight-loss programs. Programs are directly compared as to their effects on weight loss, waist circumference, and systolic and diastolic blood pressure. The review found no difference in outcomes between the programs. The first article does, however, show some small difference in some areas between programs and is helpful if you have a specific problem, such as cholesterol, that is not shifting. The second article finds that Weight Watchers has too limited data showing any improvement in heart risk above doing nothing or going to an education program. This article also suggests that Atkins may be a reasonable dietary option for patients with high cholesterol.

Hunger and satiety mechanisms and their potential exploitation in the regulation of food intake

> https://link.springer.com/article/10.1007/s13679-015-0184-5
>
> This article explains in depth why our bodies are very sensitive to negative energy balance and therefore work to put on weight but are comparatively tolerant of positive energy balance, which should send signals for us to lose the excess weight.

Lifestyle modification for obesity

> http://circ.ahajournals.org/content/125/9/1157.full
>
> This is a very good article summarizing the range of lifestyle interventions available to induce short-term weight loss. It briefly covers everything from diet to behavior modification outcomes between commercially available weight-loss programs.

A systematic review of environmental factors and obesogenic dietary intakes among adults: Are we getting closer to understanding obesogenic environments?

> http://onlinelibrary.wiley.com/doi/10.1111/j.1467-789X.2010.00769.x/full
>
> This review summarizes what factors in our environment are supposed to promote obesity, such as how close we live to a supermarket. However, the only strong evidence is living in a socioeconomically deprived area.

Weight loss diet studies: we need help not hype

http://www.thelancet.com/pdfs/journals/lancet/PIIS0140-6736(16)31338-1 .pdf

This editorial summarizes the current problems with weight-loss diets and why they are not effective in the long term.

Chapter Three

Gut microbiota composition correlates with changes in body fat content due to weight loss

http://www.wageningenacademic.com/doi/pdf/10.3920/BM2014.0104

A detailed article describing how the microorganisms in our gut change when we diet and which ones are beneficial to weight loss.

The role of gut microbiota in the development of obesity and diabetes

https://lipidworld.biomedcentral.com/articles/10.1186/s12944-016-0278-4

A general article describing the composition of gut microbiota and its effects: for example, diet, disease state, medications, and genetics.

Treating obesity and metabolic syndrome with fecal microbiota transplantation

https://www.ncbi.nlm.nih.gov/pmc/articles/PMC5045147

The gut microbiota can be altered in many ways, including probiotics (non-pathogenic organisms beneficial to the host), prebiotics (chemicals that induce growth and/or activity of commensal organisms), and fecal microbiota transplantation. This article describes fecal transplantation and how it can replace "fat"-inducing organisms with "thin" ones.

Chapter Four

Acceptance-based behavioral treatment for weight control: A review and future directions

http://www.sciencedirect.com/science/article/pii/S2352250X14000311

This paper describes acceptance-based behavioral treatments, which are a new extension to standard behavioral treatments, and it integrates some of the principles of mindfulness.

Behavioral interventions for preventing and treating obesity in adults

http://onlinelibrary.wiley.com/doi/10.1111/j.1467-789X.2007.00351.x/full

This paper adds to the information in the (following) summary paper by providing the results of the studies in a summarized way.

Behavioral treatment of obesity

https://www.ncbi.nlm.nih.gov/pmc/articles/PMC3233993

This is a well researched summary of principles of behavioral weight-loss treatment. It describes the different strategies and weighs the evidence for the short- and long-term effectiveness of behavioral therapy.

Prevalence of behavior changing strategies in fitness video games: Theory-based content analysis

http://www.jmir.org/2013/5/e81/?utm_source=feedburner&utm_medium =feed&utm_campaign=Feed%3A+JMedInternetRes+(Journal+of+Medical +Internet+Research+(atom))

This paper looks at behavioral strategies that are included in home console fitness video games. Home videos are a growing resource, and usually the press about them is poor. This paper provides a different view.

Chapter Five

Healthier U.S.: The President's health and fitness initiative. October 2003.

https://www.tib.eu/en/search/id/ntis%3Asid~oai%253Ads2%253Antis%252F 531a21c402b803781c0af16b/Healthier-US-The-President-s-Health-and -Fitness/?tx_tibsearch_search%5Bsearchspace%5D=tn

The report is quite old, but Chapter 3 is still relevant. It provides very specific information on how much activity individuals do each day and some suggestions on ways to do them. It also describes some government actions that were taken in the United States to promote fitness, for example promoting the use of parks and setting up the Healthier U.S. Web site.

National Heart, Blood, and Lung Institute. *Hearts N' Parks Community Mobilization Guide.* Bethesda, MD: National Heart, Blood, and Lung Institute, 2001. Sudocs Number: HE 20.3208:H 34/4

Provides a detailed description of what community leaders can do to get their communities active in order to fight obesity and its consequences. It contains information on how to start programs that target heart health and physical activity. Although it is targeted at community leaders, many sections are useful for individuals.

Physical activity, exercise, and physical fitness: definitions and distinctions for health-related research

https://www.ncbi.nlm.nih.gov/pmc/articles/PMC1424733

This is quite an old paper, but it clearly explains the differences between exercise, physical activity, and fitness.

U.S. Department of Health and Human Services, Surgeon General. Overweight and obesity: What you can do.

> https://its.utmb.edu/Sci_Cafe/documents/2014-Jan-Obesity/Overweight_and
> _Obesity_What_You_Can_Do_SurgeonGeneral.pdf

> This is quite a large report looking at physical activity, nutrition, and how those work together to maintain a healthy lifestyle. It contains suggestions for a graded program of physical activity.

Chapter Six

Association of pharmacological treatments for obesity with weight loss and adverse events: A systematic review and meta-analysis

> http://jamanetwork.com/journals/jama/article-abstract/2528211

> This article reviews research into combination drug treatments for obesity and compares them.

Long-term drug treatment for obesity: A systematic and clinical review

> jamanetwork.com/journals/jama/fullarticle/1774038

> This review looks at the long-term use of medications currently approved by the U.S. Food and Drug Administration to treat obesity in adults. It also covers off-label use of medications approved for other purposes that have been studied in obesity.

National Heart, Lung, and Blood Institute. *The Practical Guide: Identification, Evaluation, and Treatment of Overweight and Obesity*. Bethesda, MD: National Heart, Lung, and Blood Institute, 2000 (94 pp.). Sudocs Number: HE 20.3208:P 88

> https://www.nhlbi.nih.gov/files/docs/guidelines/prctgd_c.pdf

> *The Practical Guide* is designed to provide family physicians with tools to help them effectively manage overweight and obese adult patients. It is a little technical in places but provides an overview of treatment options in the summary.

A systematic review of anti-obesity medicinal plants—an update

> https://jdmdonline.biomedcentral.com/articles/10.1186/2251-6581-12-28

> A comprehensive article looking at a range of potential anti-obesity herbal plants including studies with *Nigella sativa*, *Camellia sinensis*, *Crocus sativus L*, Seaweed *Laminaria digitata*, Xantigen, virgin olive oil, Catechin enriched green tea, Monoselect Camellia®, Oolong tea, Yacon syrup, *Irvingia gabonensis*, Weigh-level, RCM-104 compound of *Camellia sinensis*, Pistachio, Psyllium fibre, black Chinese tea, sea buckthorn, and bilberries.

Chapter Eight

Body contour surgery in massive weight loss patients: Redefining body lift surgery and other contour deformities

https://www.intechopen.com/books/body-contouring-and-sculpting/body
-contour-surgery-in-massive-weight-loss-patients

This article contains several before-and-after pictures of successful abdominal plastic surgery to remove excess skin after major weight loss. Not for the fainthearted but heartening.

Getting back in the game after significant weight-loss

http://www.obesityaction.org/educational-resources/resource-articles-2
/general-articles/getting-back-in-the-game-after-significant-weight-loss

A motivating short article about ways to overcome barriers that still exist within us after significant weight loss. Learning to reprogram life after significant weight loss is not always easy. Many factors can negatively affect our ability to live fully and with satisfaction, and this article talks about some of them with a refreshing frankness.

Official Journal of the International Union of Aesthetic Medicine—UIME

http://beautifulmed.it/wp-content/uploads/2016/09/AESTETIC-MEDICINE
-VOL.2.pdf#page=35

This article contains a contact list with e-mail addresses for all the aesthetic surgery organizations worldwide. Very useful if you are looking for a clinician outside the United States.

Sexual functioning and obesity: A review

http://onlinelibrary.wiley.com/doi/10.1038/oby.2012.104/full

This article reviews all the current research on how sexual difficulties affect the lives of people living with obesity.

Chapter Nine

Healthy obese versus unhealthy lean: The obesity paradox

https://www.researchgate.net/profile/Carl_Lavie/publication/279030376
_Healthy_Obese_versus_Unhealthy_Lean_the_Obesity_Paradox/links
/55d522cf08ae1e65166374a1/Healthy-Obese-versus-Unhealthy-Lean-the
-Obesity-Paradox.pdf

This paper reviews the evidence about people with obesity who have no other health problems and whether they are healthy. It is termed the "obesity paradox."

Chapter Ten

Binge Eating Disorder Association
    https://bedaonline.com/understanding-binge-eating-disorder
    Provides advice and support for sufferers and their families.

Index